T0315162

CASE STUDIES

in

DIABETES

Edited by

D John Betteridge BSc MB BS PhD MD FRCP FAHA

Professor of Endocrinology and Metabolism
Division of Medicine
Royal Free and University College Medical School
London, UK

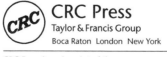

CRC Press
Taylor & Francis Group
Boca Raton London New York

CRC Press is an imprint of the
Taylor & Francis Group, an **informa** business

CRC Press
Taylor & Francis Group
6000 Broken Sound Parkway NW, Suite 300
Boca Raton, FL 33487-2742

First issued in paperback 2019

© 2003 by Taylor & Francis Group, LLC
CRC Press is an imprint of Taylor & Francis Group, an Informa business

No claim to original U.S. Government works

ISBN-13: 978-1-84184-032-1 (hbk)
ISBN-13: 978-0-367-39520-9 (pbk)

Visit the Taylor & Francis Web site at
http://www.taylorandfrancis.com

and the CRC Press Web site at
http://www.crcpress.com

Contents

Type 2 diabetes

Chronic complications

Contributors

F Javier Ampudia-Blasco
Department of Endocrinology and
Nutrition, Hospital Clínico
Universitario, Valencia, Spain

Alessandro Antonelli
Metabolism Unit, Department of
Internal Medicine and CNR Institute
of Clinical Physiology, University of
Pisa School of Medicine, Pisa, Italy

Peter H Bennett
National Institute of Diabetes and
Digestive and Kidney Diseases,
National Institutes of Health, Phoenix,
AZ, USA

Kerstin Berntorp
Department of Endocrinology, Malmö
University Hospital, Malmö, Sweden

James Best
University of Melbourne, Department
of Medicine, St Vincent's Hospital,
Fitzroy, Victoria, Australia

D John Betteridge
Division of Medicine, Royal Free and
University College Medical School,
London, UK

Poonam Bhalla
Diabetes and Endocrinology Research
Group, University Hospital Aintree,
Liverpool, UK

Sherri Blackstone
Division of Endocrinology, Diabetes,
and Metabolic Diseases, Thomas
Jefferson Hospital, Philadelphia, PA,
USA

Andrew JM Boulton
University of Manchester and
Manchester Royal Infirmary,
Manchester, UK

AC 'Felix' Burden
Heart of Birmingham Diabetes Care,
Heart of Birmingham PCT,
Birmingham, and University of
Leicester, Leicester, UK

Ian W Campbell
Medical Unit, Victoria Hospital,
Kirkcaldy, and University of
St Andrew, Fife, UK

Rafael Carmena
Department of Endocrinology and
Nutrition, Hospital Clínico
Universitario, Valencia, Spain

Alan Chait
Division of Metabolism,
Endocrinology, and Nutrition,
Department of Medicine, University of
Washington, Seattle, WA, USA

Mark Cooper
The Baker Medical Research Institute,
Central Melbourne, Victoria, Australia

Umesh Dashora
Department of Diabetes, Royal
Victoria Infirmary, Newcastle upon
Tyne, UK

Marie Degerblad
Department of Endocrinology and
Diabetology, Karolinska Hospital,
Stockholm, Sweden

Michaela Diamant
Diabetes Centre, Department of
Endocrinology, 'Vrije Universiteit'
University Medical Centre,
Amsterdam, The Netherlands

Anne Dornhorst
Department of Metabolic Medicine,
Imperial College at Hammersmith
Campus, London, UK

Michael Edmonds
Diabetic Foot Clinic, King's College
Hospital, Denmark Hill, London, UK

Gerry Fegan
Fremantle Hospital, Perth, Western
Australia

Ele Ferrannini
Metabolism Unit, Department of
Internal Medicine and CNR Institute
of Clinical Physiology, University of
Pisa School of Medicine, Pisa, Italy

Brian M Frier
Department of Diabetes, Royal
Infirmary of Edinburgh, Edinburgh,
UK

John E Gerich
General Clinical Research Center,
University of Rochester Medical
Center, Rochester, NY, USA

Lisa Hamzah
Department of Medicine, Royal Free
& University College Medical School,
The Middlesex Hospital, London, UK

Markolf Hanefeld
Centre for Clinical Studies, Technical
University of Dresden, Dresden,
Germany

Klavs W Hansen
Medicine Department M, Arhus
Kommunehospital, Arhus, Denmark

Robert J Heine
Diabetes Centre, Department of
Endocrinology, 'Vrije Universiteit'
University Medical Centre,
Amsterdam, The Netherlands

P Jean Ho
Diabetes Centre, Royal Prince Alfred
Hospital, Camperdown, NSW, Australia

Hanna Huopio
Assistant Physician, Department of
Paediatrics, University of Kuopio,
Kuopio, Finland

Serge Jabbour
Division of Endocrinology, Diabetes,
and Metabolic Diseases, Thomas
Jefferson Hospital, Philadelphia, PA,
USA

Graham Jackson
Cardiac Department, St Thomas
Hospital, London, UK

George Jerums
Endocrinology Unit and Department
of Medicine, The University of
Melbourne, Austin, and Repatriation
Medical Centre, Heidelberg, Victoria,
Australia

Ulrich Julius
Institute and Polyclinics of Clinical
Metabolic Research, University
Hospital Dresden,
Dresden, Germany

Maria Karlsson
Department of Dermatology,
Karolinska Hospital, Stockholm,
Sweden

Michael J Krimholtz
Department of Endocrinology,
Diabetes & Internal Medicine, Guy's
Hospital, King's College London,
London, UK

Wilhelm Krone
Klinik II und Poliklinik für Innere
Medizin, University of Cologne,
Cologne, Germany

Markku Laakso
Professor and Chair, Department of
Medicine, University of Kuopio,
Kuopio, Finland

James M Lawrence
Specialist Registrar in Diabetes and
Endocrinology, Royal United Hospital,
Bath, UK

Pierre J Lefèbvre
Division of Diabetes, Nutrition and
Metabolic Disorders, Department of
Medicine, University Hospital, Liege,
Belgium

Robert S Lindsay
National Institute of Diabetes and
Digestive and Kidney Diseases,
National Institutes of Health, Phoenix,
AZ, USA

Vincent McAulay
Department of Diabetes, Royal
Infirmary of Edinburgh, Edinburgh,
UK

Andrew MacIsaac
Department of Cardiology, St Vincent's
Hospital, Melbourne, Victoria, Australia

Richard J MacIsaac
Endocrinology Unit and Department
of Medicine, The University of
Melbourne, Austin, and Repatriation
Medical Centre, Heidelberg, Victoria,
Australia

Carl E Mogensen
Medicine Department M, Arhus
Kommunehospital, Arhus, Denmark

Dirk Müller-Wieland
Clinical Biochemistry, Heinrich-Heine
University of Düsseldorf, German
Diabetes Centre, Düsseldorf, Germany

Katriina Nikkilä
Department of Medicine, Division of
Diabetes, University of Helsinki,
Helsinki, Finland

John J Nolan
Endocrinology, St James' Hospital,
Trinity College Dublin, Dublin, Ireland

Stephen O'Rahilly
Clinical Biochemistry, University of
Cambridge, Addenbrooke's Hospital,
Cambridge, UK

Julia Ostberg
Department of Diabetes and
Endocrinology, University College
London Hospitals, London, UK

Petra Ott
Centre for Clinical Studies, Technical
University of Dresden, Dresden,
Germany

Philip H Passa
Department of Diabetology, Saint-
Louis Hospital, Paris, France

Andrew I Pettit
Specialist Registrar in Diabetes and
Endocrinology, Weston General
Hospital, Weston Super Mare, UK

Per L Poulsen
Medicine Department M, Arhus
Kommunehospital, Arhus, Denmark

John PD Reckless
Consultant Endocrinologist, Royal
United Hospital, Bath, UK

Gabriele Riccardi
Department of Clinical and
Experimental Medicine, Federico II
University, Naples, Italy

Martin Ridderstråle
Department of Endocrinology, Malmö
University Hospital, Malmö, Sweden

Anthony M Robinson
Consultant Endocrinologist, Royal
United Hospital, and Honorary Senior
Lecturer, University of Bath, Bath, UK

David Savage
Clinical Biochemistry, University of
Cambridge, Addenbrooke's Hospital,
Cambridge, UK

Russell S Scott
Department of Lipid and Diabetes
Research, Christchurch Hospital,
Christchurch, New Zealand

Soon H Song
c/o Medical Unit, Victoria Hospital,
Kirkcaldy, Fife, UK

Peter GF Swift
Leicester Royal Infirmary Children's
Hospital, Leicester, UK

Mehmooda Syeed
Division of Endocrinology, Diabetes,
and Metabolic Diseases, Thomas
Jefferson Hospital, Philadelphia, PA,
USA

Lisa R Tannock
Division of Metabolism,
Endocrinology, and Nutrition,
Department of Medicine, University of
Washington, Seattle, WA, USA

Andrew Taylor
Consultant Clinical Biochemist, Royal
United Hospital, Bath, UK

Roy Taylor
Department of Diabetes, Royal
Victoria, Infirmary, Newcastle upon
Tyne, UK

Merlin Thomas
The Baker Medical Research Institute,
Central Melbourne, Victoria, Australia

Stephen Thomas
King's Diabetes Centre, King's College
Hospital, Denmark Hill, London, UK

John E Tooke
Institute of Biochemical and Clinical
Science, Peninsula Medical School
Exeter, Plymouth, UK

Arno WFT Toorians
Department of Endocrinology, 'Vrije
Universiteit' University Medical
Centre, Amsterdam, The Netherlands

Elena Toschi
Metabolism Unit, Department of
Internal Medicine and CNR Institute
of Clinical Physiology, University of
Pisa School of Medicine, Pisa, Italy

John R Turtle
Department of Medicine, University of
Sydney, NSW, Australia

Olga Vaccaro
Department of Clinical and
Experimental Medicine, Federico II
University, Naples, Italy

Giancarlo Viberti
Department of Endocrinology,
Diabetes & Internal Medicine, Guy's
Hospital, King's College London,
London, UK

Peter J Watkins
King's Diabetes Centre, King's College
Hospital, London, UK

Gareth Williams
Department of Medicine, University
Hospital Aintree, Liverpool, UK

Myra Yeo
Department of Endocrinology and
Diabetes, St Vincent's Hospital,
Melbourne, Victoria, Australia

Hannele Yki-Järvinen
Department of Medicine, Division of
Diabetes, University of Helsinki,
Helsinki, Finland

Preface

Postgraduate medical education is much more structured than 30 years ago, when I embarked on a career in hospital medicine. This has tremendous advantages for the trainee physician; nevertheless, the often protracted clinical apprenticeship of former years did perhaps have the advantage of providing wide clinical experience in one's chosen specialty. Hopefully, this book will help fill some of the 'experience gap' of the shorter training period for diabetes.

I have asked international colleagues, all very experienced clinicians in diabetes, to present cases related to their clinical practice which have contributed significantly to their depth of knowledge in the subject. They discuss the educational points arising from their real-life cases and point the reader to useful references and further reading.

Clearly, the fascination of diabetes as a clinical and research interest relates not only to the disordered metabolism as a consequence of insulin deficiency and insulin resistance, but also to the protean complications of this chronic disease. Though by no means a comprehensive catalogue, the cases discussed in this volume should provide the reader with interesting insights into the diagnosis and management of many important common and some less common problems in the clinical care of patients with diabetes.

I would like to thank the colleagues and friends who have contributed to this project; there has been universal enthusiasm for it. Interested physicians continue to study and learn throughout their careers, and I have no doubt that these illustrative case reports will be of interest not only to those beginning their specialist careers, but also those well established in diabetic practice.

My publishers, Martin Dunitz, and particularly Alan Burgess, have been especially supportive of this educational project. Giovanna Ceroni, Senior Production Editor, has been of great help in putting the volume together, along with my personal assistant Jean De Luca. Finally, I am sure that my clinical colleagues would wish to thank their patients who continue to inspire them to greater efforts in clinical care and research.

D John Betteridge
London, 2003

CASE 1: A CLASSICAL CASE OF NEW DIABETES PRESENTING WITH DIABETIC KETOACIDOSIS?

Per L Poulsen, Klavs W Hansen and
Carl E Mogensen

History

A 36-year-old woman was admitted to our hospital with 2–4 month history of fatigue, polyuria, thirst, weight loss and abdominal pains. She reported no prior diseases not any familial predisposition to endocrinological diseases. She received no medication. On admission, she was hyperventilating, with nausea and vomiting, but mentally alert.

Examination and investigations

Evidence of marked dehydration was present. Blood pressure was 95/55, heart rate 104, body temperature 37.1°C, respiration 36, with a distinct smell of ketones on the breath. No focal signs of infection were evident and physical examination was otherwise unremarkable. No hyperpigmentation, alopecia, or vitiligo was observed.

Blood values were as follows: Na^+, 132 mmol/L; K^+, 6.6 mmol/L; HCO_3 , 13 mmol/L; urea, 9.7 mmol/L; glucose, 22 mmol/L; arterial pH, 7.2.

Heavy ketonuria was present.

Diagnosis

Diabetic ketoacidosis was obvious. However, marked hyponatraemia and hyperkalaemia prompted a short ACTH stimulation test which had the following outcome: p-cortisol, 159–196 nmol/L (30 min > 550 nmol/L); ACTH, 141 ng/L (9–52 ng/L). Circulating adrenal antibodies (IgG) were strongly positive. An MRI of the abdomen showed normal adrenal glands.

Treatment and outcome

Diabetic ketoacidosis was treated as usual with fluid replacement, i.v. insulin and replacement of electrolytes. In addition, 100 mg of i.v. hydrocortisone was given three times a day for the first 2 days and subsequently the dose was gradually reduced to hydrocortisone 20 + 10 mg daily and fluorocortisone 0.1 mg daily. After she had recovered from the diabetic ketoacidosis, the ACTH stimulation test was repeated, with a virtually identical outcome. Her actual dose of insulin is now Actrapid 8 + 6 + 8 units and Insulatard 14 units for the night. On this medication the patient is doing remarkably well, she is working fulltime and is now planning pregnancy. She is regularly screened for appearance of other signs of polyglandular insufficiency such as autoimmune thyroid disease, pernicious anaemia, primary hypogonadism, myasthenia gravis and coeliac disease, but as yet no signs of other autoimmune diseases are evident.

Commentary

The concept of polyglandular disease was introduced over 80 years ago by reports of patients with coexistent non-tuberculous adrenal insufficiency and lymphocytic thyroiditis. In 1926 Schmidt described the relationship between adrenal and thyroid failure with or without diabetes mellitus which has now become a syndrome recognized as Schmidt's syndrome or polyglandular syndrome type II (PGSII). The syndrome is strongly associated with the HLA alleles B8 and DR3.

What did I learn from this case?

Type 1 diabetes is associated with other autoimmune diseases. Primary adrenal insufficiency (Addison's disease) often develops insidiously. Although a rare disorder, it is more common in type 1 diabetes mellitus as part of PGSII. Recurrent hypoglycaemia despite reductions in dose of insulin is the usual presentation, but simultaneous onset of Addison's disease and diabetes mellitus has been described earlier.

How much did this case alter my approach to the care and treatment of my patients with diabetes?

Diabetic ketoacidosis is a frequent complication of diabetes which often responds well to standard routine treatment. However, a high level of attention to potential precipitating factors and coexisting diseases should be maintained and careful re-examination performed. In otherwise well-controlled patients with diabetes 'unexplainable' changes in insulin demand should always raise the suspicion of other concomitant autoimmune diseases.

Further reading

Baker JR. Autoimmune endocrine disease. *JAMA* 1997; **278**: 1931–7.

Iisalo E. Simultaneous onset of Addison's disease and diabetes mellitus. A case report. *Ann Med Intern Fenn* 1967; **56**: 37–40.

Papadopoulos KI, Hallengren B. Polyglandular autoimmune syndrome type II in patients with idiopathic Addison's disease. *Acta Endocrinol (Copenh)* 1990; **122**: 472–8.

Schmidt MB. Ein biglandulare erkrankung (nebennieren und schilddruse) bei morbus addisoni. *Verh Dtsch Ges Pathol* 1926; **21**: 212–21.

Zelissen PM, Bast EJ, Croughs RJ. Associated autoimmunity in Addison's disease. *J Autoimmun* 1995; **8**: 121–30.

CASE 2: MIXED DIABETIC KETOACIDOSIS AND HYPEROSMOLARITY

Richard J MacIsaac and George Jerums

Introduction

Traditional teaching describes two distinct hyperglycaemic emergencies which are potentially life-threatening, i.e. diabetic ketoacidosis (DKA) in young patients with type 1 diabetes and a hyperglycaemic, hyperosmolar state (HHS) in older patients with type 2 diabetes. In clinical practice, patients of varying ages can present with decompensated diabetes that is associated with concurrent DKA and hyperosmolarity, but this has been poorly documented. We discuss the case of a patient who presented with a diabetic hyperglycaemic emergency associated with mixed acidosis and hyperosmolarity that was precipitated by an infective process. The key steps in managing a hyperglycaemic emergency are also outlined.

History

A 37-year-old man, without a history of diabetes, was transported to the Emergency Department by ambulance with a decreased conscious state. A history obtained from a relative who lived with the patient revealed 2 weeks of polyuria and polydipsia, with the patient drinking large volumes of 'soft drinks'. For 3 days preceding admission he was suffering from nausea and vomiting. There were no overt symptoms of intercurrent infection, in particular the relatives could not recall the patient complaining of any mouth or jaw pain. The patient had no significant past medical history. He was not taking any medications and had no history of drug or alcohol abuse. There was no formal past history of psychiatric illnesses. However, according to his relatives the patient had not sought medical advice because he was a social recluse. On the day of admission he was found to have a depressed conscious state and an ambulance was called.

Examination and investigations

The patient had a Glasgow Coma Scale of 6/15, was profoundly dehydrated and had ketotic smelling breath. He was hypotensive (blood pressure = 105/80), tachycardic (pulse = 93/min), tachypnoeic (respiratory rate = 26/min) and hypothermic (temperature = 33°C). There were no focal neurological signs. On examination there was no evidence of a chest infection and his abdomen was soft and non-tender.

His biochemical investigations showed hyperglycaemia (glucose = 86 mM), a profound metabolic acidosis (arterial pH = 6.88 and venous HCO_3 = 7 mM), an elevated lactate level (4.5 mM), hypokalaemia (potassium = 2.2 mM), hyperosmolarity (calculated serum osmolarity = 388 mOsM, i.e. 2 × [Na + K] + urea + glucose), renal failure (creatinine = 0.55 mM), a leucocytosis (total white cell count = 16.9 × 10^9/L and neutrophil count = 14.9 × 10^9/L) and mild ketonuria (urine analysis = 1 plus ketones). There was no evidence of myocardial ischaemia on his electrocardiogram and no evidence of infection on chest X-ray.

Diagnosis

A diagnosis of DKA with a concurrent hyperosmolar state was made.

Treatment and outcome

Given the patient's depressed conscious state, he was intubated and transferred to the intensive care unit. At the time of intubation poor dental hygiene was noted.

A nasogastric tube plus a central venous and arterial line were inserted. Intravenous hydration and potassium replacement were commenced followed by an insulin infusion (5 units/h). Although the patient was oliguric careful potassium replacement was commenced as haemofiltration was started shortly after admission. Before the initiation of haemofiltration his lactate level had decreased to 1.2 mM. The patient was slowly warmed and empirical intravenous antibiotics in the form of cefotaxime and metronidazole were administered. A computerized tomography (CT) scan of the brain revealed mild cerebral oedema but no focal pathology. Approximately 18 h after admission the patient's biochemical parameters were glucose, 30 mM; potassium, 4.6 mM; arterial pH, 7.35; and creatinine, 0.32 mM. His serum glucose levels were slowly reduced and when they had declined to 15 mM an infusion of dextrose was commenced. After 48 h the patient's glucose levels were ranging between 10 and 17 mM on an insulin infusion of 1–2 units/h. Prophylaxis for deep vein thrombosis in the form of subcutaneous heparin was started but this was stopped after 2 days due to the development of thrombocytopenia (platelet count = 16 × 10^9/L).

After the patient was warmed, a temperature of 38°C was noted. Three days after admission he remained febrile despite the above antibiotics. There was no significant bacterial growth from urine or blood cultures. He was then referred to the Oral and

Maxillofacial Surgery Unit for assessment of his oral cavity as a possible source of the persistent fever. Examination revealed a 2-cm abscess associated with the lower left 5th tooth. Five millilitres of brown pus were drained with a needle and culture of this specimen revealed a mixed infection of dental origin. Given this finding, ampicillin was added to the intravenous antibiotic regimen. On day 5 after admission he was taken to theatre for a full dental clearance, surgical drainage of the abscess and antral washout under general anaesthesia.

The day after the procedure the patient's conscious state improved and he was extubated. His plasma glucose levels were stable, the white blood cell and platelet counts were within the normal range and he was afebrile. The patient was then transferred to a general ward. As he was tolerating a soft oral diet he was subsequently treated with subcutaneous insulin in the form of lispro insulin with meals and isophane insulin nocte. His intravenous antibiotics were stopped and he was placed on a 10-day course of amoxycillin and clavulanic acid. After psychiatric review a diagnosis of agoraphobia was made. He received intensive physiotherapy for a severe left foot drop (a recognized complication of severe DKA) and was discharged 20 days after admission.

Commentary

Although it is not well documented, patients often present with hyperglycaemic emergencies that are associated with concurrent acidosis and hyperosmolarity. Indeed, one study has demonstrated that 33% of presentations for diabetic hyperglycaemic emergencies across a wide range of age groups have a mixed state of acidosis and hyperosmolarity.[1] Recently we also demonstrated that 30% of admissions for hyperglycaemic emergencies are characterized by a mixed acidotic and hyperosmolar state.[2]

Classifying patients with diabetes and acidosis on the basis of hyperosmolarity has practical applications. Hyperosmolarity may be a risk factor for mortality, although this has not been a consistent finding.[1,3] Our patient had a depressed conscious state at presentation and it has been demonstrated previously that the degree of hyperosmolarity and not acidosis is best correlated with conscious state.[4] It has been suggested that if a patient has ketoacidosis, without significant hyperosmolarity and presents with a depressed mental state, another cause to account for their conscious state should be searched for, i.e. a stroke, overdose, meningitis or another metabolic derangement.[5] Thus, assessing the plasma osmolarity of diabetic patients with acidosis may also help to identify cases that require a more intensive approach to their management. Our patient most likely developed hyperosmolarity because of a delay in presentation and because he was drinking large amounts of glucose-containing fluids. The majority of patients with DKA do not develop significant hyperosmolarity because the gastrointestinal effects of acidosis, i.e. nausea and vomiting, usually result in an early presentation.

It is not uncommon for patients with previously undiagnosed diabetes to first present with DKA. However, in patients with a history of diabetes the main precipitants of DKA include non-compliance with their insulin therapy and infections.[6] Most DKA patients who receive appropriate therapy make an uneventful recovery, but fatalities do occur. Our experience over the period 1986–1999 has found mortality rates of 1.2% for DKA alone, 5.3% for mixed DKA and HHS and 17% for HHS alone[2] (see Figure 1). We also found that when the associations between age, category of diabetic emergency, serum osmolarity and various other biochemical parameters were assessed by logistic regression analysis, age and the degree of hyperosmolarity were found to be the most powerful predictors of a fatal outcome. In particular, patients aged >65 years presenting with a serum osmolarity >375 mOsM were at greatest risk. However, in a multivariate analysis only age emerged as a significant independent predictor of mortality (p<0.01). No death was attributable solely to the metabolic derangement of acidosis or hyperosmolarity. Our patient had evidence of cerebral oedema on CT and while cerebral oedema is the main cause of mortality in paediatric patients it has rarely been reported to cause death in adult patients with DKA.[7] Patients with a hyperosmolar state are often placed on thrombotic prophylaxis as there is some evidence to suggest that it may improve outcome.[8] In this case the patient's heparin therapy was stopped after 2 days due to the development of thrombocytopenia.

Infective processes, delays in diagnosis and a delay in seeking medical intervention have all been implicated as potentially reversible factors in fatal cases.[6] Acute dento-alveolar abscess complicating DKA is a rare event; there are

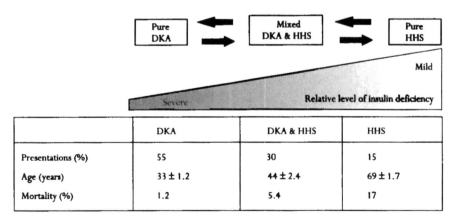

	DKA	DKA & HHS	HHS
Presentations (%)	55	30	15
Age (years)	33 ± 1.2	44 ± 2.4	69 ± 1.7
Mortality (%)	1.2	5.4	17

Figure 1 *The spectrum of hyperglycaemic emergencies.[5] The presentation profiles and outcomes of 312 admissions for hyperglycaemia associated with diabetic ketoacidosis (DKA) and/or a hyperglycaemic, hyperosmolar state (HHS).[2]*

only four reported cases in the literature.[9,11] Chest and urinary tract infections are the most common causes but, as illustrated by this report, dento-alveolar abscess should also be considered. Another condition that should always be included in the differential diagnosis of DKA associated with an oral or maxillofacial infection is murcormycosis. This is a rare but often fatal complication of DKA.[12] Our patient was improving clinically after drainage of the dental abscess and with the addition of ampicillin to his antibiotic regimen and hence this diagnosis was considered unlikely in this particular case.

Recently, a position statement on the management of hyperglycaemic crises has been released by the American Diabetes Association.[13,14] The key diagnostic procedures include a history and physical examination with special attention to 1) patency of the airway, 2) mental status, 3) cardiovascular and renal status, 4) sources of potential infection and 5) state of hydration. The therapeutic goals consist of 1) correcting fluid and electrolyte imbalances, 2) decreasing serum glucose and ketone levels and 3) identifying and treating precipitating factors. It is worth noting that the majority of patients with hyperglycaemic emergencies present with a leucoytosis and this does not necessarily indicate the presence of an infective process per se. However, in the above case potentially more attention could have been paid to examining the oral cavity as a source of sepsis after the patient was stabilized.

The case also emphasizes the importance of measuring serum potassium levels and if necessary starting replacement therapy before commencing an insulin infusion. Without potassium replacement the administration of insulin or bicarbonate may result in fatal hypokalaemia. Potassium replacement should also be considered in the context of renal status. This is usually not commenced before it is established that a patient is producing urine. Our patient was oliguric and had acute renal failure, but careful potassium replacement was commenced as his serum potassium was low and haemodialysis was initiated soon after presentation.

Serum lactate levels are frequently moderately elevated in patients with DKA (i.e. < 5 mM) and as in this particular case declined quickly with intravenous hydration. Poor tissue perfusion due to hypovolaemia is usually responsible for elevated lactate levels in DKA. However, consideration should always be given to other possible causes of an elevated lactate level, e.g. cardiac ischaemia, septic shock, bowel infarction and metformin therapy in patients with type 2 diabetes. Our patient did not receive bicarbonate therapy. Administration of bicarbonate to patients with an arterial pH 6.9–7.1 does not alter the course or outcome of a hyperglycaemic emergency and its effects in patients with an arterial pH < 6.9 are not known.[14]

In summary, pure DKA or HHS represent the extremes of the spectrum of hyperglycaemic emergencies and often patients present with elements of both conditions (Figure 1). Although patients can have profound metabolic disturbances most will make an uneventful recovery if careful attention is paid to the management steps outlined above.

References

1. Wachtel TJ, Tetu-Mouradjian LM, Goldman DL, Ellis SE, O'Sullivan PS. Hyperosmolarity and acidosis in diabetes mellitus. *J Gen Intern Med* 1991; **6**: 495–502.

2. MacIsaac RJ, Lee LY, McNeil KJ, Tsalamandris C, Jerums G. Influence of age on the presentation and outcome of acidotic and hyperosmolar diabetic emergencies. *Intern Med J* 2000; **32**: 379–85.

3. Pinies JA, Cairo G, Gaztambide S, Vazquez JA. Course and prognosis of 132 patients with diabetic non ketotic hyperosmolar state. *Diabetes Metab* 1994; **20**: 43-8.

4. Fulop M, Tannembaum H, Dreyer N. Ketotic hyperosmolar coma. *Lancet* 1973; **2**: 635–9.

5. Siperstein MD. Diabetic ketoacidosis and hyperosmolar coma. In: Karam JH, ed. *Diabetes Mellitus: Perspectives on Therapy* – Endocrinology and Metabolism Clinics of North America, Vol. 21, No. 2. Philadelphia: WB Saunders, 1992; 415–31.

6. Fishbein H, Palumbo PJ. Acute metabolic complications of diabetes. In: *Diabetes in America*, 2nd edn. Betheseda, MD: National Institutes of Health Publication No 95-1468, 1995; 283–91.

7. Edge JA. Cerebral oedema during treatment of diabetic ketoacidosis: are we any nearer finding a cause? *Diabetes Metab Res Rev* 2000; **16**: 316–24.

8. Rolfe M, Ephraim GG, Lincoln DC, Huddle KRL. Hyperosmolar non-ketotic diabetic coma as a cause of emergency hyperglycaemic admission to Baragwanath Hospital. *S Afr Med J* 1995; **85**: 173–6.

9. Moskow DE. Dentoalveolar abscess complicated by diabetic ketoacidosis in a previously undiagnosed diabetic: report of case. *J Conn State Dent Assoc* 1988; **62**: 126–9.

10. Shahgoli S, Shapiro R, Best JA. A dentoalveolar abscess in a paediatric patient with ketoacidosis caused by occult diabetes mellitus: a case report. *Oral Surg Oral Med Oral Pathol Oral Radiol* 1999; **88**: 164–6.

11. Chandu A, MacIsaac RJ, Smith ACH, Bach LA. Diabetic ketoacidosis secondary to dento-alveolar infection. *Int J Maxillofac Surg* 2002; **31**: 57–9.

12. Hendrickson RG, Olshaker J, Duckett O. Rhinocerebral mucormycosis: a case of a rare, but deadly disease. *J Emerg Med* 1999; **17**: 641–5.

13. American Diabetes Association. Hyperglycaemic crises in patients with diabetes mellitus. *Diabetes Care* 2001; **24**: 154–61.

14. Kitabchi AE, Umpierrez GE, Murphy MB et al. Management of hyperglycaemic crises in patients with diabetes. *Diabetes Care* 2001; **24**: 131–53.

CASE 3: RECURRENT VOMITING AND DIABETIC KETOACIDOSIS IN A TYPE 1 DIABETIC FEMALE

Ian W Campbell and Soon H Song

History

A 35-year-old female with a 16-year history of type 1 diabetes mellitus was admitted with a 3-day history of vomiting. Her diabetic control had been poor for many years, with glycated haemoglobin levels of 11–12% (lab range 4.4–7.0%). There were prolonged periods of default from the outpatient clinic. Relevant past medical history showed that there had been 2 previous episodes of severe diabetic ketoacidosis (DKA) in the previous 2 years, both associated with vomiting. This intermittent vomiting was first investigated two years earlier by upper gastrointestinal endoscopy, which showed a large amount of food debris in the

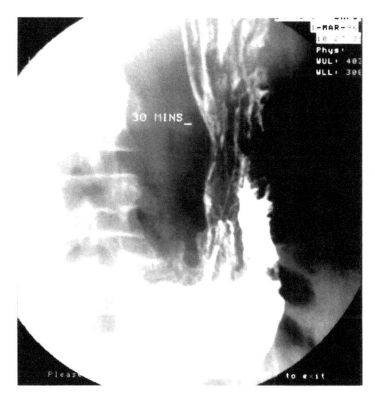

Figure 1

Barium meal examination showing gross gastric and duodenal dilatation delaying the emptying of barium from the stomach.

stomach with no evidence of gastric outlet obstruction. Barium meal examination at this time demonstrated gross gastric dilatation with decreased peristaltic activity (see Figure 1) in keeping with a diagnosis of gastric atony ('gastroparesis diabeticorum'). In the intervening 2 years a further two gastroscopies were done because of recurrent vomiting (not associated with DKA) and these showed similar findings.

Examination and investigation

The patient looked unwell, was afebrile and appeared dehydrated clinically with Kussmaul (acidotic) respiration. The pulse was regular at 120 beats/min; the patient was hypotensive, BP 90/60 mmHg. There was no obvious clinical source of infection.

Plasma glucose was 55 mmol/L, Na 145 mmol/L, K 5.0 mmol/L, urea 10.8 mmol/L, creatinine 144 µmol/L. Arterial blood gases showed pH 7.18, bicarbonate 8 mmol/L, base excess −23 mmol/L, PO_2 (on air) 15.9 Kpa and PCO_2 of 0.9 Kpa. The full blood count showed a haemoglobin of 15.1 g/dl, a neutrophilia with WBC 24.9×10^9/L and platelets of 513×10^9/L. The blood cultures were negative. MSU was negative. Chest X-ray and routine ECG were both normal.

Treatment and outcome

The DKA was treated aggressively with intravenous normal saline-containing fluids and a sliding-scale i.v. low dose insulin regime; when the plasma glucose fell to 14 mmol/L, 5% dextrose-containing fluids replaced saline. Appropriate additions of potassium chloride were added to the saline and dextrose solutions according to the serial biochemistry results. Over the subsequent 24 h the patient's clinical status improved and the acute metabolic decompensation resolved with a plasma glucose of 6.7 mmol/L, Na 150 mmol/L, K 3.7 mmol/L, bicarbonate 24 mmol/L, urea 8.6 mmol/L, creatinine 99 µmol/L. The arterial pH was 7.46, base excess −0.2, PO_2 12.0 Kpa.

The patient made a full recovery from the DKA. In view of the recurrent vomiting due to gastric atony a detailed history and examination was performed to assess for diabetic complications. Background diabetic retinopathy was present. Urinalysis was negative for protein (Labstix) and albumin excretion was normal at 8 mg/L (microalbumin range 20–200 mg/L). Peripheral pulses were readily felt and clinically there was no macrovascular disease. There was evidence of a peripheral sensory neuropathy with loss of light touch sensation and pinprick appreciation to mid-calf level in both lower limbs; absent knee and ankle jerks were noted, as was the loss of vibration sense at both big toes and ankles.

On further enquiry the patient admitted to light-headedness and dizziness. Postural hypotension was confirmed with supine BP of 90/60 mmHg falling to 70/40 mmHg on standing. A normal short Synacthen test excluded Addison's disease. For the previous 2 years she had noticed intermittent episodes of watery diarrhoea with faecal incontinence in keeping with diabetic diarrhoea. Several stool samples showed no infection.

Several simple cardiovascular tests for diabetic autonomic neuropathy (DAN) were performed as shown in Box 1.

Box: 1 Tests for diabetic autonomic neuropathy

Tests reflecting parasympathetic activity

1. Heart rate response to Valsalva manoeuvre: an abnormal result of 1.0 was obtained
2. Heart rate response during deep breathing: an abnormal response of < 10 beats per minute was found
3. Immediate heart rate response to standing (30:15 ratio): an abnormal result of 0.9 was noted.

Tests reflecting sympathetic function

4. Blood pressure response to standing: abnormal systolic fall of 30 mmHg was seen
5. Blood pressure response to sustained hand grip: an abnormal result of < 10 mmHg was noted.

The postural hypotension improved with fludrocortisone 0.1 mg daily. The gastric atony symptoms were controlled with a combination of metoclopramide 10 mg tds and erythromycin 500 mg qds. The diabetic diarrhoea went into 'spontaneous remission' although occasional faecal incontinence is still a problem. The patient's diabetic control on twice-daily Velosulin and Insulatard insulins is erratic, with glycated haemoglobin levels running at 12–14%.

Learning points

• The ketosis and acidosis of DKA can cause vomiting but recurrent vomiting itself may precipitate DKA. Inadequate carbohydrate intake together with increasing concentrations of 'stress' hormones (catecholamines, cortisol and glucagon) can cause increased lipolysis, ketosis and acidosis.

- DKA can cause *acute* gastric dilatation due to electrolyte disturbances, especially those involving potassium and magnesium. Gastric emptying will return to normal once the acute metabolic decompensation has been corrected. This acute gastric dilatation has to be differentiated from the *chronic* gastric atony due to diabetic autonomic neuropathy.
- Gastric atony due to DAN is often asymptomatic but it should be suspected when other severe autonomic nervous system complications are present such as postural hypotension or diabetic diarrhoea.
- Diabetic control may be very erratic with recurrent hypoglycaemia as a result of a delay in the passage of food from the stomach to the small intestine. Hyperglycaemia itself may aggravate the delayed gastric emptying. When the gastric stasis is severe, acute bouts of hiccups, nausea and vomiting may occur, resulting in DKA.
- Further complications of gastric atony include poor absorption of oral medications, some of which may be required. Drugs that can delay gastric emptying such as tricyclic antidepressants (with anticholingeric activity), β-adrenergic agonists and morphine, L-dopa should be avoided if possible. Hypokalaemia and hypomagnesaemia should be corrected and any hypothyroidism treated appropriately.
- Pro-kinetic drugs such as dopamine agonists, metoclopramide or domperidone, together with a motilin receptor agonist, e.g. erythromycin, are the treatments of choice. Cisapride was withdrawn in July 2000 because of reports of prolonged QT interval associated with ventricular arrhythmias and sudden death. When the vomiting is intractable and unresponsive to drugs, surgery such as gastro-jejunostomy or a Roux-en-Y jejunal loop procedure with partial gastrectomy may help, but results are variable.
- Where the gastric atony is gross, diagnosis can be made with simple barium meal examination showing a grossly dilated stomach with diminished or absent peristalsis and delayed emptying of barium. In less severe cases the barium meal may be normal and the evaluation of gastric emptying may be determined by radionuclide gastric emptying scans using solid and liquid meals with radio-opaque markers.

Approach to future management

- The patient was instructed to eat small and regular meals. If vomiting occurred she was instructed to check her urine for ketones and where there was moderate or heavy ketonuria, further instruction was given for the patient to present early to hospital for intravenous fluids and insulin to abort any severe DKA.
- The various medical, and occasionally surgical, treatments of DAN are purely symptomatic. They in no way alter the natural history and poor prognosis of

this complication of diabetes. The case presented had symptoms of gastric atony, diabetic diarrhoea and postural hypotension together with abnormal tests of cardiovascular reflex function. Such patients have a 3-year mortality of almost 50%. Sudden, apparently unexplained deaths may occur in patients with DAN, who seem to be prone to cardiorespiratory arrest.

In this case and with similar cases the goal of insulin treatment should be to keep the patient free of hyperglycaemic symptoms on the one hand and avoid hypoglycaemia on the other. Any further glycaemic benefit should be regarded as a 'bonus'.

Further reading

Diabetic ketoacidosis

Kitabchi AE, Kreisberg RA, Umpierrez GE et al. Management of hyperglycaemic crisis in patients with diabetes. *Diabetes Care* 2001; **24**: 131–53.

Lebovitz HE. Diabetic ketoacidosis. *Lancet* 1995; **345**: 767–72.

Diabetic autonomic neuropathy and gastric atony

Campbell IW. Diabetic autonomic neuropathy. In: Tattersall RB, Gale EM, eds. *Diabetes: Clinical Management*. Edinburgh: Churchill Livingstone, 1990: 307–20.

Ewing DJ, Campbell IW, Clarke BF. The natural history of diabetic autonomic neuropathy. *Q J Med* 1980; **49**: 245–7.

Kong M-F-S-C, Macdonald IA, Tattersall RB. Gastric emptying in diabetes. *Diabetic Med* 1996; **13**: 112–19.

Stacher G. Diabetes mellitus and the stomach. *Diabetologia* 2001; **44**: 1080–93.

CASE 4: MAINTAINING TIGHT GLYCAEMIC CONTROL DURING INTERMITTENT HIGH-DOSE PREDNISOLONE ADMINISTRATION DURING TYPE 1 DIABETIC PREGNANCY

Umesh Dashora and Roy Taylor

Little has been published on how tight blood glucose control may be maintained when high dose steroid therapy management has to be commenced. This matter is of particular relevance in pregnancy when blood glucose levels in the normal range are sought. Increase in steroid doses can lead to progressive increase in blood glucose, the levels rising into the range of 12–25 mmol/L. We present the case of a pregnant woman with type 1 diabetes and severe hyperemesis requiring high dose steroid therapy in whom tight control of diabetes was maintained with appropriate modifications in insulin dose.

History

A 35-year-old midwife with a 20-year history of type 1 diabetes developed nausea and vomiting at 5 weeks gestation in her second pregnancy. Blood glucose control has been tightened prior to conception and her last pre-pregnant HbA1c was 7.5%. At booking HbA1c was 7.1% and a scan confirmed 6 + 2 weeks gestation. Over the next 11 weeks vomiting occurred several times each day with associated weight loss.

By 17 weeks she was too weak to undertake everyday activities. HbA1c at that time was 5.8% and insulin dose as Actrapid (AR) 18, 16, 14 and Insulatard (IT) 40. She was started on prednisolone 10 mg tid. Insulin was simultaneously increased to AR 22, 22, 18 and IT 50. She reported an immediate cessation of vomiting and nausea. At 19 + 1 week gestation she was much improved with no nausea and had returned to full activities. Weight had increased by 0.5 kg. HbA1c was 5.9%. Median value of home blood glucose monitoring (HMBG) from a computerized record of the period from 15 week to 17 week pregnancy showed readings before meals and at bedtime to be 3.3, 6.1, 11.8 and 6.3 mmol/L. Corresponding values immediately after steroids were started were 14.3, 14.6, 12.6 and 11.3 mmol/L. Insulin dose was further increased to AT 30, 26, 24 and IT 66 units to optimize blood glucose control in the face of markedly increased food consumption. Prednisolone dosage was tapered to zero over 13 weeks and insulin doses were reduced appropriately. HbA1c remained between 5.8% and 6.1%.

Off steroids, the nausea and vomiting returned. There was no postural fall of BP. Prednisolone was restarted as 10 mg tid at 31 + 5 weeks. At the time of restarting steroids, insulin dose was increased from AR 24, 24, 24 + IT 56 units to AR 34, 34, 36 + IT 72 units (an increase of 48%). The HMBG record remained stable throughout the steroid treatment. The median values of blood glucose before meals and before bedtime before steroid treatment were 8.3, 13, 5.4 and 6.5 mmol/L respectively. After steroid treatment they remained 8.5, 9.1, 5.0 and 6.5 mmol/L for corresponding points of time. HbA1c was 6.0% at this time. The symptoms responded dramatically quickly once again. She remained stable for the rest of her pregnancy, the prednisolone dose was reduced to 20 mg daily over the remaining 4 weeks.

At 36 + 5 weeks she was admitted for planned induction of labour. Within 2 hours of delivery the nausea stopped completely. The rate of insulin infusion was decreased by 50% at the end of the second stage of labour as per the Newcastle protocol,[1] plasma glucose remaining stable between 3 and 5 mmol/L. Steroid dose was tapered over 2 days. She was discharged on AR 16, 16, 14 + IT 40 units, this being similar to the pre-pregnancy insulin requirements.

Commentary

This case illustrates some very important lessons with regard to the management of diabetes in all patients requiring high dose steroid therapy for any reason. An increase of approximately 40% in insulin dose is required in this situation, and the increased dose should be given at the same time as steroid therapy is commenced. Both patient and staff have to be reassured that the apparently large increase in insulin dosage will not cause hypoglycaemia when given at the same time as the first dose of oral prednisolone. This was shown to be appropriate on two occasions in the case reported. On the first occasion, an initial increase of 31% was undertaken as a cautious step in view of the anorexia, and on the second the increase of 48% was appropriate.

The role of steroids in the management of severe hyperemesis gravidarum has now been established.[2-4] However, steroids disturb diabetes control. The effect of glucocorticosteroids is usually rapid and persists only for the duration of therapy. In a study measuring blood glucose response to alternate day prednisone dosing, patients exhibited hyperglycaemia in the afternoons of the days when the steroids were given.[5] Blood glucose levels normalized throughout the next day (the day off steroids). This rapid onset of steroid-induced insulin resistance is striking, and out of keeping with the widely assumed mechanism of action of steroid hormones in interacting with nuclear receptors and changing gene expression.[6]

A hallmark of diabetic pregnancy is the increase in the insulin requirement between 18 and 30 weeks of gestation.[7][9] The underlying trend can be seen in Figure 8.1. The placenta-driven rise in anti-insulin hormones over the last two trimesters[1][7][9] is believed to be responsible. Consistent with this, the insulin resistance disappears within as soon as the placental circulation shuts down after the second stage of labour. The average increase in insulin requirements in pregnancy is 40%, commencing around 18 weeks gestation.[1] In our patient the additive effects of pregnancy and steroids in bringing about the need for increased insulin dose was evident (see Figure 1).

The need for immediate and calculated increase in insulin at onset of high dose steroid administration is not widely appreciated. An increase in insulin dose of approximately 40% works well even in the complicated situation of pregnancy with tight blood glucose control.

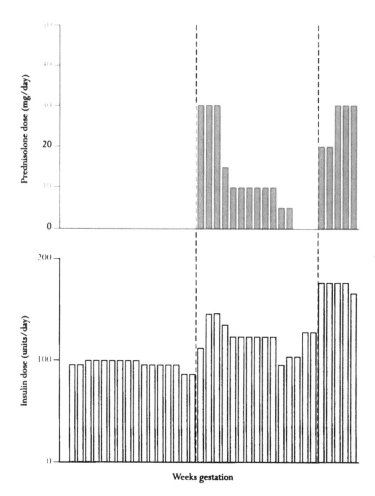

Figure 1 The two courses of prednisolone each required an immediate increase in insulin dose. The more cautious approach to increasing insulin dosage in view of the lack of food intake which was adopted for the first course was shown not to be required. Overall blood glucose control was maintained despite the high dose steroids and the change in eating pattern.

19

References

1. Carron Brown S, Kyne-Grzebalski D, Mwangi B, Taylor R. Effect of management policy upon 120 type 1 diabetic pregnancies: policy decisions in practice. *Diabetic Med* 1999; **16**: 573–8.

2. Taylor R. Successful management of hyperemesis gravidarum using steroid therapy. *Q J Med* 1996; **89**: 103–7.

3. Nelson-Piercy C, Fayers P, de Swiet M. Randomised, double-blind, placebo-controlled trial of corticosteroids for the treatment of hyperemesis gravidarum. *Br J Obstet Gynaecol* 2001; **108**: 9–15.

4. Moran P, Taylor R. Management of hyperemesis gravidarum: the importance of weight loss as a criterion for steroid therapy. *Q J Med* 2002; **95**: 153–8.

5. Greenstone MA, Shaw AB. Alternate day corticosteroid causes alternate day hyperglycemia. *Postgrad Med J* 1987; **63**: 761–4.

6. Grunfled C, Baird K, Van Obberghen E, Kahn CR. Glucosteroid-induced insulin resistance in vitro: evidence for both receptor and post-receptor defects. *Endocrinology* 1981; **109**: 17–23.

7. Steel JM, Johnstone FD, Home R, Mao JH. Insulin requirements during pregnancy in women with type I diabetes. *Obstet Gynecol* 1994; **83**: 253–8.

8. McManus RM, Ryan EA. Insulin requirements in insulin-dependent and insulin-requiring GDM women during final month of pregnancy. *Diabetes Care* 1992; **15**: 1323–7.

9. Langer O, Anyaegbunam A, Brustman L, Guidetti D, Levy J, Mazze R. Pregestational diabetes: insulin requirements throughout pregnancy. *Am J Obstet Gynecol* 1988; **159**: 616–21.

CASE 5: POSTPARTUM GRAVES' DISEASE IN A TYPE 1 DIABETIC WOMAN

Rafael Carmena and F Javier Ampudia-Blasco

History

A white woman was diagnosed with type 1 diabetes at the age of 21. She was started on diet and insulin (0.4 U/kg/day) and 4 months later became pregnant (White class B). She was referred to our department because of poor diabetic control. Pertinent laboratory tests at that time were: HbA1c 8.6%; basal C-peptide 0.04 ng/ml (normal range 0.8–4.0) and anti-GAD titre 14.5 UI/ml (normal < 1.0).

During pregnancy the insulin dose was increased to 0.9 U/kg/day administered in two doses. HbA1c was kept below 7.4%, and total weight gained was 10 kg. She delivered a healthy 3200-g male after 36 weeks by caesarean section. During the following 2 years she was treated at another clinic with conventional insulin therapy (Humulin 20:80 at 0.6 U/kg/day, 20 U breakfast and 10 U dinner) and remained in good general condition. Her HbA1c ranged from 6.4% to 9.0%. At age 37 she was again referred to our department because of a second, unplanned pregnancy (White class C).

Her HbA1c was 8.3%. She was placed on intensified insulin therapy with three boluses of regular insulin (10 U before breakfast and lunch and 7 U before dinner) and 14 U NPH at dinner (0.9 U/kg/day) and her HbA1c during pregnancy was kept between 5.9% and 6.6%. She was very compliant with the insulin regimen but gained 20 kg in weight. After 38 weeks of gestation an elective caesarean procedure and a tubarian ligature were performed. A healthy 3700-g male was born. She was treated with bromocriptine to suppress lactation and remained on intensified insulin therapy with three boluses of regular insulin and NPH before dinner.

Four months after delivery she felt increasingly nervous and developed anxiety, fatigue, palpitations and heat intolerance, and lost 14 kg in the ensuing 4 months. She was referred to our Department for evaluation of possible hyperthyroidism.

Examination and investigations

Her weight was 47 kg (BMI 19.2 kg/m^2), blood pressure 110/70 mmHg and resting heart rate 98 bpm. There was diaphoresis and fine tremor in both hands, lid stare but no evidence of infiltrative ophthalmopathy or dermopathy. The thyroid gland was firm and only moderately enlarged, without bruit. Relevant biochemical tests were: free T4 3.14 ng/dl (normal 0.85–1.70) and TSH < 0.002 mcU/ml (normal 0.50–4.00); TSH receptor antibodies (TSI) 28 UI/ml (normal 0–10). Thyroid echography showed a gland that was normal in size, structure and morphology. A thyroid technetium (Tc) scan (Figure 1) showed diffuse uptake. TSH assay in the infant was normal.

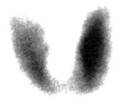

Figure 1 *Thyroid scan showing diffuse uptake of technetium.*

Diagnosis

The diagnosis of Graves' disease was based on the presence of hyperthyroidism, suppressed TSH, elevated free T4 and titre of TSI, and diffuse uptake of technetium by the thyroid.

Treatment and outcome

Initially, the patient was treated with propranolol (up to 160 mg/day) and methimazole (up to 40 mg/day), which were tapered down to a maintenance dose of 10 mg/day of methimazole. One year later 5 mCi of radioactive iodine was given, and additional therapy with thionamides could be stopped 3 months after that. One year after the radioactive iodine the patient remains free of symptoms and no substitutive therapy with levothyroxine has been necessary so far.

Commentary

Graves' disease is an autoimmune disease caused by IgG thyroid-stimulating antibodies (TSI), which bind to and activate the thyrotropin receptor on thyroid cells, and results in hyperthyroidism. The disease is more prevalent in women, with an annual incidence of around 0.5 per 1000.

Susceptibility to Graves' disease is determined by genetic, environmental and endogenous factors. The mechanisms responsible for the activation of T and B lymphocytes against the thyrotropin receptor are unknown. Type 1 diabetes, a paradigm of autoimmune disease, not infrequently coexists with hypothyroidism or hyperthyroidism.[1] Furthermore, up to 20% of type 1 diabetics show elevated titres of thyroid autoantibodies. The underlying abnormality responsible for this polyglandular autoimmunity is most likely a defect in T suppressor cell function, but there is evidence that aberrant expression of HLA DR antigens also plays an important role in the pathogenesis of these disorders.

Autoimmune thyroid disease is usually suppressed during pregnancy and is exacerbated in the postpartum period.[2] New-onset autoimmune thyroid disease occurs in up to 10% of women after delivery, and an increased risk of 6.5 of developing Graves' disease within 1 year after delivery has been reported.[3] Up to 60% of Graves' patients in the reproductive years give a history of postpartum onset,[4] as in the case of the patient presented. Moreover, recurrence of hyperthyroidism in the postpartum period in patients with Graves' disease, who were in clinical remission before and during pregnancy, has been described.[3] The significant weight gain and lack of symptoms of hyperthyroidism militate against Grave's disease being present during pregnancy in our patient, although no definite proof exists, as no thyroid function tests were performed.

What did I learn from this case?

The natural history of Graves' disease in pregnancy is characterized by aggravation in the first trimester, amelioration in the second half, and recurrence in the year following delivery.[5] If possible, it is best to avoid thyroid surgery during pregnancy because of the possible induction of premature labour. Antithyroid agents (thionamides) at the lowest possible dose are the therapy of choice during pregnancy. Propylthiouracil is preferred to methimazole because of the greater transplacental passage of the latter.[6] The postpartum period has been associated with a greater frequency of onset (as in our case), recurrence, or exacerbation of thyrotoxicosis resulting from Graves' disease.[3] After an initial treatment with thionamides, radioactive iodine is a safe therapeutic approach to control hyperthyroidism in Graves' patients in the postpartum period.[7] In women of child-bearing age, pregnancy should not be contemplated until one year after radioactive iodine therapy.

Postpartum Graves' disease must be distinguished from postpartum thyroiditis.[3,4] Postpartum thyroiditis often appears during the first 3 months after delivery. The incidence is variable, ranging from 1.9 to 16.7%. Frequently, after a transient and brief thyrotoxic phase characterized by a low uptake of technetium, a subsequent more lasting phase of hypothyroidism supervenes. Thyroid function abnormalities are usually mild and transient. Hypothyroidism becomes permanent in only a small proportion of cases. In contrast, women who experience thyrotoxicosis from Graves' disease in the postpartum period usually initiate the clinical picture after the first 3 months, as in the patient reported here. Characteristically, Graves' patients show a high diffuse thyroid uptake of technetium and can have an elevated titre of antibodies to TSH receptor.

How much did this case alter my approach to the care and treatment of my patients with diabetes?

Thyroid disorders are the most common endocrine diseases, after diabetes, during and after pregnancy. In particular, pregnant women with type 1 diabetes have an increased risk of developing postpartum thyroiditis and Graves' disease. Because of this, it is recommended that thyroid function should be checked in diabetic women during pregnancy and especially after delivery[1]. If thyroid function tests become altered in the first 3 months after delivery, a probable diagnosis of postpartum thyroiditis should be excluded. On the other hand, thyroid dysfunction diagnosed beyond that period usually indicates Graves' disease or autoimmune hypothyroidism (Hashimoto's thyroiditis).

References

1. Eisenbarth GS, Ziegler AG, Colman PA. Pathogenesis of insulin-dependent (type I) diabetes mellitus. In: Kahn CR, Weir GC (eds). *Joslin's Diabetes Mellitus* 13th edn. Philadelphia: Lea & Febiger, 1994; 219–23.

2. Jansson R, Dahlberg PA, Winsa B, Meirik O, Sawenberg J, Karlsson A. The postpartum period constitutes an important risk for the development of clinical Graves' disease in young women. *Acta Edocrinol (Copenh)* 1987; 116: 321–5.

3. Glinoer D. Thyroid disease during pregnancy. In: Braverman LE, Utiger RD (eds.). *Werner and Ingbar's The Thyroid* 8th edn. Philadelphia: Lippincott, Williams & Wilkins, 2000; 1013–27.

4. Davies TF. The thyroid immunology of the postpartum period. *Thyrid* 1999; 9: 675–84.

5. Mestman JH. Hyperthyroidism in pregnancy. *Endocrinol Metab Clin North Am* 1998; 27: 127–49.

6. Momotani N, Noh JY, Ishikawa N, Ito K. Effects of propylthiouracil and methimazole on fetal thyroid status in mothers with Graves' hyperthyroidism. *J Clin Endocrinol Metab* 1997; 82: 3633–6.

7. Lazarus JH, Ludgate ME. Prevention and treatment of postpartum Graves' disease. *Ballieres Clin Endocrinol Metab* 1997; 11: 549–60.

CASE 6: A HISTORY OF SURVIVAL IN A NATURAL SURVIVOR

Anne Dornhorst

The case I have chosen to present raises the question we too rarely ask, namely 'why do some patients do so well while others do so badly'? I strongly believe that if we could answer this question at a molecular level, it would provide pharmacological options to prevent or minimize many diabetic complications. Until we know the answer, we should stop taking the credit for all good outcomes, while attributing all the bad ones to poor diabetic care or poor patient compliance. The case described below highlights our inability to accurately predict the future, while illustrating how the medical dogma and pessimism of its day can profoundly affect patients' daily lives and their expectations and fears for the future.

History

The patient is a now elderly man who developed type 1 diabetes at the age of 8 and has lived through the medical advances and achievements of the twentieth century requiring little more than the initial discovery of insulin itself. This 76-year-old man with a 20-year history of cigarette smoking is essentially free of diabetic microvascular complications. For the cynics among you, he has not got MODY, but true type 1 diabetes, confirmed by a lifetime dependency on insulin and a history of diabetic ketoacidosis. He admittedly received the very best of care throughout his early life from the most eminent and prestigious physicians of the day, and his family's affluence and influence undoubtedly facilitated access to this care. However, this is not why the patient has done so well; in fact the dietary regime handed down to him by RD Lawrence would be ridiculed today by most opinion leaders in the field, and the bovine and porcine insulins he received for most of his diabetic life would be considered inferior to our present-day highly purified genetically engineered insulins. His 20-year smoking history would certainly have received more self-righteous disapproval from today's diabetic medical establishment than 50 years ago, and while not endorsing cigarette smoking, perhaps we should modify the tone of our judgemental predictions when it comes to frightening our patients with the inevitability of amputations and heart attacks if they choose not to heed to our advice, as there remains an element of luck in all this, or at least genetic susceptibility, which is currently beyond our control or understanding.

I was privileged to meet this gentleman a year ago in a diabetic clinic immediately after seeing a patient who had developed type 1 diabetes at the age of 3, and although now extremely well in his 40s he had a relatively bad family history of heart disease. By the end of my consultation with this patient I had persuaded him to start an aspirin, a statin and an ACE inhibitor in the belief that I was reducing his long-term morbidity and mortality. I have little doubt I terrified him of his own mortality in the process. My next patient was Mr GG, the 76-year-old gentleman who seriously questioned, not only how I had treated the previous patient, but also my overall outlook on diabetic morbidity and mortality.

Mr GG had developed diabetes in 1933 at the age of 8, while in Cornwall staying with his grandparents, who were in loci parentis while his father (a colonial civil servant) and his mother were abroad. He presented with a 2-week history of unquenchable thirst and was diagnosed quickly by an astute local general practitioner on a urine test. He was referred locally and within the week had started twice-daily insulin injections using a glass syringe and steel needles. It was recommended that he saw Dr RD Lawrence in London, who he did indeed consult with and was subsequently seen by him during his school holidays throughout his childhood and adolescence, however he received most of his medical care from school doctors and local GPs. RD Lawrence provided him with the basic management and dietary principles by which Mr GG continues to live his diabetic life today. Sixty-eight years on he still restricts his carbohydrate intake along the principles of carbohydrate exchanges initially taught to him in 1933. Lawrence provided social as well as medical support, as exemplified by him being instrumental in getting this young diabetic patient accepted into a boarding school. During the pre-war years most boarding schools were extremely reluctant to take on the responsibilities for insulin injections and the supervision of the diet prescribed. These restricted educational choices in turn limited access to further education and career opportunities. His parental expectations for their eldest son to attend Winchester College followed by Oxbridge and a career in the Diplomatic Service were dealt a fatal blow the day the Cornish general practitioner diagnosed diabetes, a day when all hopes and expectations switched to the more sanguine goal of survival into adulthood. Despite one hospital admission, with diabetic ketoacidosis at 10 years old, he remained well and achieved this first milestone with relative ease. His survival through puberty incarcerated in minor public boarding schools with no free access to food outside designated mealtimes (when it was strictly rationed) was undoubtedly helped by his highly, no doubt physiologically programmed, instinctive primordial food-scavenging behaviour which during pubescence overcame any guilt associated with pilfering. During these years he was able to feed a hunger as intense as the thirst he initially experienced at the onset of his diabetes. At 18 years he served in the Home Guard and became an articled clerk in a firm of solicitors. After a number of positions with London City firms, he finally settled in a career of conveyancing, probate and trust. All safe career choices made to accommodate his diabetes and the medical uncertainties of his future. During this time he continued to receive the best private medical care of the day and remained rigidly wedded to the Lawrence diet of carbohydrate exchanges. By the age of 35 years, already more than a decade beyond his own childhood perceived life expectancy, he married and subsequently had three healthy children. By the age of 45 years, completely fit and without any diabetic complications, he first attended an NHS diabetic outpatient clinic, since when all his diabetic care has alternated between teaching hospital diabetic outpatient clinics and his own general practitioner. His general health has remained extremely good and he has minimal diabetic retinopathy, with less than five microaneurysms in each eye. He did, however, require bilateral cataract extractions in his early seventies, which may, or may not, have been diabetic in their aetiology. He has latterly developed mild, but stable, peripheral vascular disease. Nevertheless, he can still walk half a mile or more a day on the flat, which is no mean achievement for someone who had smoked over 20 cigarettes a day until the age of 40.

Commentary

So, the case I present to you is a man with 68 years' experience of living with diabetes in the twentieth and twenty-first centuries, who remains remarkably well. He remains thankful for the help and advice given to him by RD Lawrence and the medical fraternity in general, which he intends to acknowledge in a legacy to Diabetes UK. But I believe his greatest legacy is that he shows us that there is an answer to an as yet undefined scientific question(s), that when understood will help us prevent diabetic microvascular and possibly other complications in our patients.

Case 7: Type 1 diabetes in adolescents is still a dramatic disease

Philip Passa

History

Ten years ago, John was 15 years old when we met for the first time in my office. Type 1 diabetes was diagnosed at the age of 7 and since then had been poorly controlled with NPH insulin, 20 units before breakfast and dinner.

Physical examination was normal, his height was 1 m 74, he weighed 69 kg. Blood pressure values were 110/70 mmHg. Casual capillary blood glucose in the outpatient clinic was 19 mmol/L and HbA1c 11.5% (normal value < 6%). Despite this very poor metabolic condition, he had no complaint at all. He did not do well at school, but was very fond of rock and roll music; he was very keen to become a music star.

During his first hospitalization for 5 days, no microvascular complication was detected, the insulin regimen was shifted to regular insulin, 18 units in the morning, 14 units at lunch and NPH insulin, 25 units before dinner. His diet was normal, apart from a reduction in sugars.

Over the following 6 years, he regularly attended the outpatient clinic, as a smiling, nice-looking adolescent; HbA1c was always > 10%. He never experienced severe ketoacidosis or a hypoglycaemic episode. He claimed that he was in fair condition with high blood glucose values, while he felt fatigue and dizziness when 'by accident' his blood glucose was near normal.

At the age of 21, he was an unemployed musician. HbA1c reached 12%, and denied omitting insulin injections, even during overnight disco-parties. Despite the absence of detectable retinopathy, nephropathy and neuropathy, he was clearly and precisely informed about the risk of severe vascular complications related to his long-term hyperglycaemic condition.

For the next 4 years, he failed to attend the clinic. Six months ago, he came back to the hospital, as an emergency, for severe loss of visual acuity. His physical examination was still normal, apart from blood pressure values of 155/90 mmHg. HbA1c was 11.5%. Severe proliferative retinopathy (Figure 1) was present in both eyes, with vitreous haemorrhages. The 24-hour proteinuria was 3 g, plasma creatinine was within normal values. He then agreed that for many years, insulin injections were performed only once or twice a day, to prevent hypoglycaemia during the daily music sessions with his band.

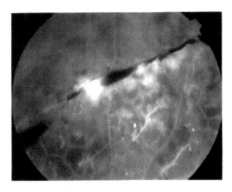 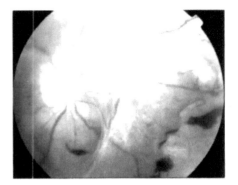

Figure 1 *Severe diabetic retinopathy.*

John is now a very compliant type 1 diabetic patient. However, despite improved glycaemic control, tight blood pressure control using a combined diuretic and an ACE inhibitor, cryocoagulation and vitrectomy, his visual acuity did not improve significantly and is still less than 1/6 in both eyes.

Commentary

John's story is a dramatic failure of health care delivery in a centre mainly devoted to the prevention of diabetic micro- and macro-angiography. In 2001, blindness due to type 1 diabetes, at the age of 25, should be prevented. For some patients, commonly used approaches to information and education are grossly inadequate and do not help the fight against a devastating chronic disease. The development of new, original types of education is mandatory. In France, diabetic patients are 100% reimbursed by the Sécurité Sociale for all the expenses caused by their disease. For those who failed to benefit from periodical examination, should such a reimbursement be interrupted? The early diagnosis of incipient retinopathy and/or nephropathy is useful to prevent blindness or end-stage renal failure, with all their human and financial consequences.

During the last few months (using the computer at the clinic) I decided to send a letter and to propose an appointment for all type 1 diabetic patients aged < 40 years who do not attend the clinic regularly. The number of such patients is large, much more than expected, and most of them have HbA1c values > 8%. During a 30-minute visit, a more aggressive treatment and surveillance are proposed.

The current rapid increase in type 2 diabetes prevalence is of major concern for diabetologists; however, they have to remember that poorly controlled type 1 diabetic patients are still at risk of developing severe, premature complications.

Case 8: Type 1.5 diabetes

John J Nolan

History

In July 1999, a 34-year-old sales executive sought further advice on his diabetes. Recently, his fasting glucose had been poorly controlled at 8–12 mM and postprandial values were 10–16 mM. He complained of intermittent balanitis. He was not currently taking medication. Two years previously, at age 32, diabetes was diagnosed at a routine pre-employment medical examination. He was treated with diet and metformin, with good initial control. He weighed 80.5kg (BMI 25.4) when diagnosed in 1996 compared with 73 kg in 1999. Blood pressure was normal. A first cousin had insulin-treated diabetes and another was recently diagnosed with type 2 diabetes. He had no relevant past medical history.

Examination and investigations

He was of medium build and normotensive. There were no features to suggest a secondary form of diabetes. His liver edge was palpable. There was no clinical evidence of diabetes complications.

Fasting plasma glucose, 12.7 mM; HbA1c 8% (upper limit of normal 6.9%); total cholesterol, 5.86 mM (LDL cholesterol, 3.71 mM; triglycerides, 1.45 mM; HDL cholesterol, 1.48 mM). Renal, liver and bone biochemistry were normal, thyroid function was normal. Albumin to creatinine ratio was 0.6 mg/mM (normal). Ferritin 243 (normal). Fasting C-peptide, 1.0 µg/L (0.2–3.2). Fasting insulin, 4.4 uU/ml. GAD antibodies were strongly positive.

Diagnosis

Immune-mediated insulin-deficient diabetes of slow onset (type 1.5 diabetes, or slow onset type 1 diabetes, or latent autoimmune diabetes of adulthood, LADA).

Treatment and outcome

I explained the laboratory findings to the patient and indicated that he would probably eventually need insulin to achieve good glucose control. This was not immediately necessary, however, and we commenced a trial of glipizide 5 mg pre-breakfast. Formal dietary consultation was arranged. After 3 months, he remained well, with morning glucose averaging 8 mM and late evening glucose often above 10 mM. Daytime control during working hours remained satisfactory. His glipizide was increased to 5 mg bd and later to 10 mg bd and then 20 mg am with 10 mg pm. He gained weight (3 kg) and his HbA1c improved from 8% to 7.3%. Because his evening glucose continued to be poorly controlled, his glipizide dose was increased to 20 mg bd.

As part of a research protocol, and with his informed consent, he underwent an intravenous glucose tolerance test (having discontinued his glipizide for 2 weeks before the study). This confirmed basal insulin secretion with no significant first phase response to glucose, and normal insulin sensitivity (see Figure 1). Because of continued sub-optimal glycaemic control on glipizide 20 mg bd, it was decided to introduce intermediate-acting insulin at bedtime, in combination with daytime glipizide. The starting dose was 5 U Insulatard. This improved his fasting glucose, but evening control remained poor. He was then increased to Insulatard bd (3U pre-breakfast, 7U pre-dinner). His glipizide was reduced to 10 mg bd and his insulin modified to Insulatard 5U pre-breakfast, and Mixtard 30, 8U pre-dinner, because of poor post-dinner control. On this regime, he improved with HbA1c 6.7%.

At this most recent review, he was very well, with no unwanted hypoglycaemia and excellent glycaemic control (HbA1c 6.2%) on the following regime: Insulatard 4U pre-breakfast, glipizide 10 mg bd, Mixtard 30, 7–9 U pre-dinner, depending on self monitored glucose.

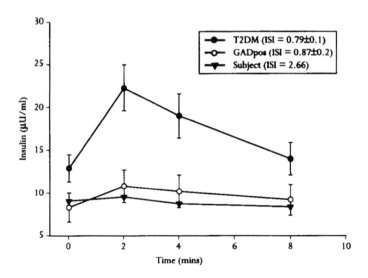

Figure 1 *Acute insulin response to glucose (AIRg) in a series of patients with (closed triangles) and without (closed circles) GAD antibodies, and in the case described here (open circles). Insulin sensitivity for each given in brackets.*

Commentary

The clinical presentation and history of progression of this man's diabetes is interesting. He has clear and quite florid evidence of altered immunity with respect to his islet cells. Despite this, he presented with an indolent form of 'type 1.5' diabetes, managing to be reasonably compensated for nearly 5 years without the addition of exogenous insulin. For much of this period, he took either no medication or low-dose sulphonylureas. He followed a fairly liberal diet without any formal exercise regime. He continued to have detectable basal C-peptide, and responded to glipizide. The main difficulty was his overnight basal control and his late evening post-dinner control. The unusual combination of the short-acting sulphonylurea with intermediate-acting insulin pre-breakfast and a pre-mixed soluble and intermediate acting insulin pre-dinner has allowed him to achieve tight glycaemic control, with normal HbA1c.

What did I learn from this case?

The clinical categories of type 1 and type 2 diabetes are often insufficient physiological explanations for cases presenting in clinical practice. This patient continued to have residual insulin secretion for several years, but did not have typical phenotypic features of type 2 diabetes. He had a high titre for GAD antibodies. Genetic tests for MODY or other rare genotypes were not yet conducted in his case. These analyses are expensive and are not generally performed outside the research setting. In this and similar cases of what can best be described as type 1.5 diabetes, a balance must be struck between long-term glycaemic control (and the risk of diabetes complications) and the risks and benefits of insulin in a patient who does not absolutely require insulin. In this man's case, an incremental regime could be designed to fit his relative degree of insulin deficiency, without putting him at undue risk of hypoglycaemia. He currently enjoys excellent control and quality of life.

How much did this case alter my approach to the care and treatment of my patients with diabetes?

We know that about 13% of patients presenting with type 2 diabetes have antibodies against components of the pancreatic insulin secretory system. These GAD-positive type 2 patients (also referred to as LADA, or sometimes as type 1.5 diabetes) were originally thought to be stereotypical type 1 patients with typical type 1 phenotype except for their more gradual loss of insulin secretion. In fact, our experience has been different. Many of these patients have a type 2 diabetes phenotype, with obesity and insulin resistance. What these patients clearly show, however, is a selective loss of first phase insulin secretion, compared with age- and weight-matched subjects with antibody-negative type 2 diabetes (see Figure 21.1). This patient fits this category quite well, although he is young and of medium build. Knowledge of a patient's insulin secretory reserve as well as islet antibody status, together with an estimate of their insulin sensitivity, can add valuable information the process of customizing diabetes treatment. Diabetes in this sub-group of patients appears to have a different pathogenesis. In the future, it may be possible to limit or ablate the immune damage in these slow-onset patients by immunization or gene therapy. With current treatment options, earlier customized insulin therapy or combination therapy is certainly effective.

Further reading

Isomaa B, Almgren P, Henricsson M et al. Chronic complications in patients with slowly progressing autoimmune type 1 diabetes (LADA). *Diabetes Care* 1999; 22: 1347–53.

Tuomi T, Carlsson A, Li H et al. Clinical and genetic characteristics of type 2 diabetes with and without GAD antibodies. *Diabetes* 1999; 48: 150–7.

Yousif O, O'Gorman DJ, O'Donghaile D, Gasparro D, Pacini G, Nolan JJ. GAD positive type 2 diabetes: insulin resistance with a pronounced defect in first phase insulin secretion. *Diabetes* 2001; 50 (Suppl 2): A428.

Zimmet P, Turner R, McCarty D, Rowley M, Mackay I. Crucial points at diagnosis. Type 2 diabetes or slow type 1 diabetes. *Diabetes Care* 1999; 22 (Suppl 2): B59–64.

CASE 9: EVALUATING THE DEGREE OF DIABETES CONTROL

Pierre J Lefèbvre

History

Born in May 1964, Philip was found to be diabetic in June 1989. At the time of diagnosis, he had lost 6–7 kg, had polyuria and polydipsia, his blood glucose was over 60 mmol/L and ketonuria was present. He was HLA DR4 and islet cell antibodies were present (ICA+). He was considered to have autoimmune type 1 diabetes and treated with insulin (combination of NPH and regular insulin twice a day). I saw him first in November 1989. At that time, he weighed 55.5 kg and his height was 172 cm; the body weight deficit was about 10 kg. Physical examination was otherwise normal. Non-fasting blood glucose was 9.5 mmol/L and HbA1c was 6.8%. I sent him back to his usual physician.

Philip came to see me again 1 year later. He was on 14 U of insulin twice a day, and had lost another 3.5 kg. He presented me with a diary in which most blood glucose values ranged between 5 and 8 mmol/L. Surprisingly, a 2-h pp. glucose at the laboratory gave a value of 18 mmol/L and HbA1c was 16.2%. For the next few months, such a marked discrepancy between the data of blood glucose monitoring in the patient's handbook and the laboratory data persisted, despite several calibrations and changes of the glucometer. The patient was finally given a new blood glucose meter, with an in-built memory of which he was not aware. Table 1 shows some of the blood glucose data obtained.

Further analysis revealed that over a period of 28 days, 55 blood glucose values were recorded in the patient's handbook, while only 44 were recorded in the glucometer memory, thus 11 values were 'invented'. Out of the 44 determinations performed, 21 were concordant in both the notebook and the meter memory, 1 out of 44 was 'improved' from low to higher values and 22 out of 44 were modified from high to lower values.

We decided not to inform the patient of our findings, re-emphasized the importance of metabolic control, provided a new glucometer and requested more frequent visits. Insulin doses were progressively increased, normal body weight was slowly recovered and since 1995, HbA1c levels ranged between 6.5% and 8% with compatible blood glucose values both at the laboratory and in the patient's handbook. Several months later, the patient spontaneously recognized having cheated with this home blood glucose monitoring for more than 1 year and appreciated our patience. We told him that we were convinced of his cheating but did not tell him the glucometer memory story. Were we right?

Table 1 Blood glucose data (mg/dl) from patient's handbook and the glucometer memory

Date	Time	Patient's handbook	Glucometer memory
30 Sept	9 h 30	188	188
	21 h 00	243	243
1 Oct	7 h 00	125	199
	21 h 00	108	108
2 Oct	8 h 00	85	214
	21 h 00	100	100
3 Oct	7 h 00	110	211
	21 h 00	122	Not done
4 Oct	7 h 00	105	Not done
	21 h 00	195	281
5 Oct	7 h 00	125	162
	21 h 00	101	101

Commentary

The major issue in this case is the discrepancy between the values of blood glucose obtained by the patient's monitoring and listed in his handbook and those of the HbA1c measured in the laboratory.

We suggest the following attitude:

1. Make sure that the discrepancy is indeed real by repeating laboratory measurements, particularly HbA1c. Such was the case in our patient.

2. If the discrepancy is confirmed, first consider the possibility that HbA1c levels are falsely elevated. As reviewed by Kolaczynski and Goldstein[1] and Schnedl et al.[2] falsely elevated HbA1c levels are observed with haemoglobin variants such as HbF, HbG and other negatively charged haemoglobins, as well as in other numerous conditions (e.g. uraemia (carbamylation of Hb), alcoholism, lead poisoning, elevated plasma triglycerides, iron-deficiency anaemia, post-splenectomy, hyperbilirubinaemia, opiate addiction and chronic aspirin therapy). All these causes were excluded in our patient.

3. Consider the possibility of malfunctioning of the glucometer device. This is easily checked by repeated calibration or by changing the device. This was done in our case.

4. Confront the values of blood glucose indicated in the handbook with those of the memory of the glucometer. We decided to do this without informing the patient of the presence of a memory in the glucometer. One may argue the appropriateness of this attitude. We came to it after months of follow-up and numerous and lengthy discussions with the patient, explaining the problem we had in not understanding the source of the discrepancy. When we were

convinced of the patient's cheating, we decided not to disclose the glucometer memory issue and we gradually gained the confidence of the patient, obtained a progressive increase in the daily insulin doses, a progressive gain in the body weight and a major improvement of the overall health status of the patient. Five years have passed now and data recorded in the handbook are concordant with those, including HbA1c, obtained in the laboratory. The patient spontaneously recognized the cheating and appreciated out attitude.

Learning points

Cheating with the data of home blood glucose monitoring is probably not unusual.[3,4] It has been reported to occur more frequently in children and adolescents.[5] We have described a strategy to tackle this problem, based on patience and perseverance. The strategy paid in the long-term management of the patient reported here.

References

1. Kolaczynski JW, Goldstein BJ. Glycated hemoglobin and serum proteins as tools for monitoring. In: Alberti KGMM, Zimmet P, De Fronzo RA, eds. *International Textbook of Diabetes Mellitus*, 2nd edn. Chichester: J. Wiley & Sons, 1997: 1046–66.

2. Schnedl WJ, Liebminger A, Roller RE, Lipp RW, Krejs GJ. Hemoglobin variants and determination of glycated hemoglobin (HbA$_{1C}$). *Diabetes Metab Res Rev* 2001; **17**: 94–8.

3. Citrin W, Ellis CJ, Skyler JS. Glycosylated hemoglobin: a tool in identifying psychological problems? *Diabetes Care* 1980; **3**: 563–4.

4. Mazze RS, Shamoon H, Pasmantier R et al. Reliability of blood glucose monitoring by patients with diabetes mellitus. *Am J Med* 1984; **77**: 211–17.

5. Ernould C, Graff MP, Bourguignon JP. Incidence of 'cheating' in diabetes children and adolescents. In: Laron Z, Galatzer A, eds. *Psychological Aspects of Diabetes in Children and Adolescents*. Pediatric and Adolescent Endocrinology, Basel: Karger, 1982: 43–6.

CASE 10: ALLERGY TO HUMAN INSULIN — TREATED WITH PORK INSULIN IN A VEGETARIAN

AC 'Felix' Burden

History

A man, employed as a local Government Officer, presented with poorly controlled diabetes in 1997 at the age of 47, having had diabetes since 1990. His height was 1.66 m, weight 87 kg and HbA1c 8.5%.

He found exercise difficult because of congenital problems with his knees and a painful back. He had profuse diarrhoea on his metformin therapy (850 mg three times daily). He had paraesthesiae in his feet. His blood pressure was elevated at 142/80 mmHg. An eye examination had been performed recently and was normal. Vibration sense was present and he had normal peripheral pulses. His total cholesterol was 4.2 and triglycerides 1.4, serum creatinine was normal with no proteinuria.

After discussion with him I changed therapy with reinforced diet, reduced his metformin to 500 mg twice a day, with breakfast and evening meal, and added gliclazide with increasing dosage. On this, his HbA1c remained elevated at 8.1% after 3 months on maximum dosage, but his diarrhoea had improved. I suggested to him, therefore, that he should try insulin therapy.

I changed him to a combination of isophane and soluble insulin using isophane (as Humulin I™) 20 units twice a day, and soluble insulin (as Humulin S™) 8 units with the evening meal as predicted from the insulin requirement study by Holman and Turner.[1] His tablets were stopped.

He then developed angina, and needed a bypass graft. Following this, he re-attended. His tests had improved quite markedly, but he complained of very painful injection sites and examination of the sites demonstrated erythematous swelling. The pain on injection was immediate after injecting insulin and he described the pain as being like a wasp sting.

I tried a change of manufacturer, but continuing on isophane and soluble insulin, this time using Human Actrapid™ and Human Insulatard™. This initially appeared to resolve his allergy. Three months later his HbA1c was tolerable at 7.1%, but he had redeveloped markedly painful injection sites with evidence of erythema.

I assumed his problem might be from cresol or from protamine. I accordingly changed him to Human Monotard™ insulin, because this has phenol as a preservative and zinc rather than cresol as a retardant. However, there was no improvement and temporarily we changed him back to tablets.

I then admitted him for insulin allergy testing. The responses at 0.5, 1 and 24 hours were as shown in Table 1.

Table 1 Individual responses in area of erythema (in mm) to a variety of insulin preparations

	Time (h)		
	0.5	1	24
Substance tested			
Histamine (positive control)	20	18	0
Saline (negative control)	0	0	0
Human insulin	3	3–4	0
Porcine insulin	0	0	0
Bovine insulin	9	7	0
Paraben	0	0	0
Phenol	0	0	0
Metacresol	10	9	5
Zinc	5	0	0
Isophane	0	0	0
Protamine	9	9	0

Commentary

These are obviously complex results, but I discussed them fully with the patient, and explained the results. It appeared that he had responses to human soluble or regular insulin; he reacted to metacresol as preservative, but not phenol or paraben. He also reacted to zinc and protamine. However, it appeared that isophane insulin itself, despite being made up of various chemicals to which he was allergic, did not give an allergic response. I also explained that he did not react to pork insulin. My advice, therefore, was that he needed insulin in order to control his diabetes, but the insulin needed to be pork insulin, which would allow the use of soluble insulin.

This was a difficult issue, because he was a Hindu, and did not eat pork or other meats for religious reasons. However, he agreed with me that since he needed insulin for control of his diabetes, it was likely that pork insulin was suitable, and that he should try it. In his own words, 'most religions do not approve of damaging one's health by avoidance of food stuffs'.

Following the initiation of therapy with Pork Insulatard™ in the morning and Pork Mixtard™ in the evening, his symptoms of insulin allergy resolved, and his diabetic control became reasonable (HbA1c 6.8%).

Learning points

This case illustrates one of the difficulties of controlling type 2 diabetes. It illustrates the need for inspection of insulin injection sites; it illustrates the value of analysing the allergy using one of the commercially available allergy testing kits. Finally it illustrates the need for doctor–patient discussion about culturally sensitive subjects such as diet, and medication, and that the use of unusual insulin regimes can be of benefit.

Reference

1. Holman RR, Turner RC. A practical guide to basal and prandial insulin therapy. *Diabetic Med* 1985; **2**: 45–53.

CASE 11: A CASE OF TYPE 1 DIABETES TREATED WITH CSII WITH PROGRESSIVE DECREASE OF INSULIN REQUIREMENT AND SEVERE HYPOGLYCAEMIC EPISODES

Markolf Hanefeld and Petra Ott

History

The 33-year-old patient was referred to the metabolic ward because of unpredictable hypoglycaemic episodes despite continuous reduction of insulin dosage during pump treatment in previous months.

He had a family history of type 2 diabetes (mother and grandmother). His own diabetes was diagnosed at the age of 29 when he developed a coma. Before he came to the acute care unit, he had lost 10 kg in weight. After recovery he was treated with twice mixed insulin for 2 years by his GP and during that time gained 4 kg in weight. Thereafter because of increasingly labile glucose levels, a brittle diabetes was assumed and the treatment regimen was changed to ICT without a smoothing effect of his excessive 'peak and valley' glucose profile. Therefore, he was referred to our diabetes clinic. At this time, at the age of 31, his weight was 78 kg and his height 184 cm. His clinical examination resulted in no pathological findings; blood pressure was 110/70 mmHg. His blood glucose levels during the first 24-hour profile fluctuated between 2.2 and 20.3 mmol/L. The insulin treatment was 8/3/8 units regular insulin before breakfast, lunch and dinner, respectively, and 14 IU NPH insulin at bedtime with 23 bread units over the day (Table 1), HbA$_{1C}$ 6.9%, C-peptide basal < 0.1 nmol/L. Routine laboratory tests inclusive of albuminuria showed no abnormalities. Despite intensified self-control to adapt insulin dosage, a sufficient smoothing of insulin excursions could not be achieved; therefore, an insulin pump therapy was started (Table 2).

The fasting period to examine the basal rate was conducted unobtrusively. Only a blood glucose decrease of 6 mmol/L during a 30-minute 100 W ergometry was noted.

At the age of 33 years the patient was hospitalized again. Repeated, partially severe hypoglycaemias were observed, which could not be treated by the patient

Table 1 Plasma glucose, carbohydrate intake and insulin dosage – a daily course

Time	PL glucose (mmol/L)	CU	Insulin
7.00	3.8	5	8 IU H-Hoechst
9.00	4.1	5	
11.00	2.2	5	3 IU H-Hoechst
14.00	11.3		
15.45	2.4	3	
17.00	3.1	4	8 IU H-Hoechst
19.30	1.5	2 CU additional	
21.00	4.8	1	14 IU Basal-H-Hoechst
0.00	20.3		
3.00	17.4		

Table 2

Time	Base rate	PG time/value	Bolus	CU	IU/CU
0–1	0.4	0.00/5.1			
1–2	0.5				
2–3	0.6				
3–4	0.7	3.00/4.1			
4–5	0.7				
5–6	0.8				
6–7	0.9				
7–8	1	7.15/3.9	0.5	5	0.1
8–9	0.8				
9–10	0.5	9.00/7.7	1.0	5	0.2
10–11	0.4	10.30/7.7			
11–12	0.5	11.00/9.4	2.0	5	0.2
12–13	0.5				
13–14	0.6	14.15/8.3			
14–15	0.6	15.00/6.0	1.0	4	0.25
15–16	0.7				
16–17	0.8	17.15/10.4	2.5	4	0.6
17–18	0.8				
18–19	0.6				
19–20	0.4				
20–21	0.5				
21–22	0.5	21.00/8.7			
22–23	0.5				
23–24	0.4				
Total	14.7		7	22	

himself. Since the patient was well educated, with 6–8 blood glucose self-determinations daily and bolus insulin corrections corresponding to the actual blood glucose values and the planned carbohydrates intake, insufficient compliance could be excluded as a cause of the problem. At the time of hospitalization a newly developed vitiligo of the neck and extremities was observed. Blood pressure was 120/80 mmHg; no other clinically pathological findings were detected. The body weight was 81 kg.

At the patient admission, the following parameters were determined: sodium, potassium, creatinine, ALAT, ASAT, AP, GGT, bilirubin, cholesterol, HDL-cholesterol, triglycerides, red blood cell sedimentation and blood cell count, as well as urine sediment and microalbuminuria. There were no pathological findings. The HbA1c value was 7%.

The instability of glycaemia was confirmed under ward conditions (Table 3). On the third day of hospitalization the patient developed a severe hypoglycaemia

Table 3

Time	Base rate	PG time/value	Bolus	CU	IU/CU
0–1	0.3	0.00/13.2	1.5		
1–2	0.5				
2–3	0.5				
3–4	0.6	3.00/7.8			
4–5	0.7				
5–6	0.7				
6–7	0.7				
7–8	0.5	7.00/12.8	3.5	5	0.5
8–9	0.4				
9–10	0.4	9.00/14.5	2		
10–11	0.3	10.00/4.9	0.5	3	0.2
11–12	0.2				
12–13	0.2	12.00/2.5		5	0.4
13–14	0.4	13.30/8.5	2		
14–15	0.4				
15–16	0.5	15.00/3.2	1	4	0.4
16–17	0.6				
17–18	0.6	17.15/6.6	1.5	4	0.4
18–19	0.7				
19–20	0.7				
20–21	0.5				
21–22	0.3	21.20/8.1			
22–23	0.3				
23–24	0.3				
Total	10.8		10	21	

(blood glucose of 1.4 mmol/L) after physical activity (30-minute walk), which was treated by the intravenous administration of glucose. Despite the adjacent intake of 5 additional bread units, the blood glucose values during the daily profile remained below 5 mmol/L. Similar blood glucose profiles were reported by the patient in his previous medical history.

Diagnostic investigation of the hormonal cause of this insufficiency of the counter-regulatory system was carried out. The following parameters were determined: ACTH, 1047 pg/ml (9–52 pg/mL); cortisol, 1.8 μg/dL (6–30 μg/dL); cortisol in 24h-urine, 23 mg/d (46–131 mg/d); antibodies against adrenal cortex, 1: 10; FT3, 3.1 ng/L (2.6–5.1 ng/L); FT4, 1.2 ng/dl (1.9–1.8 ng/dl); TSH, 4.9 μIU/ml (0.23–3.8 μIU/ml); MAK: 504 U/L. Normal values of LH, FSH, testosterone, prolactin, IGF1 and parathormone were observed. Thus, a pluriglandular insufficiency type 2 with diabetes mellitus type

Table 4

Time	Base rate	PG time/value	Bolus	CU	IU/CU
0–1	0.3				
1–2	0.4				
2–3	0.5				
3–4	0.6	3.00/6.8			
4–5	0.7				
5–6	0.8				
6–7	0.9				
7–8	0.8	7.10/7.9	5	5	1.0
8–9	0.7				
9–10	0.6	9.15/4.1	1.5	3	0.5
10–11	0.5				
11–12	0.4	11.30/3.8	2	5	0.5
12–13	0.4				
13–14	0.4				
14–15	0.5	14.00/10.2	1		
15–16	0.6	15.00/9.4	2	4	0.5
16–17	0.6				
17–18	0.7				
18–19	0.8	18.00/6.1	3	4	0.8
19–20	0.8				
20–21	0.7				
21–22	0.5	21.30/7.8		1	
22–23	0.4				
23–24	0.3				
Total	13.3		14.5	22	3.3

1, manifest adrenal cortex insufficiency and a latent hypothyrosis (Hashimoto thyroiditis) and vitiligo were diagnosed.

After starting a replacement treatment with hydrocortisone (12.5–5–5 mg/d – with a normal cortisol elimination) and corresponding adjustment of the insulin pump therapy, a satisfactory blood glucose control without a tendency to hypoglycaemia was obtained (Table 4).

Commentary

In the retrospective observation of this case, at the first hospitalization there was already an indication of the existence of a pluriglandular insufficiency. Thus, along with the very low insulin demand, a clear decrease of the blood glucose level under conditions of physical activity existed 2 years before the diagnosis. Also the course of body weight changes was interesting in this respect – 4 years after the start of insulin therapy there was an insufficiency of 3 kg body weight at HbA1c values till maximally 7% and sufficient, even higher carbohydrate intake, from the weight before the manifestation of diabetes. Vitiligo is also a clear indication of the existence of pluriglandular insufficiency, which was detected during hospitalization.

Unclear blood glucose fluctuations as well as unusual alterations of the insulin demand in type 1 diabetic patients could be considered as an indication of the existence of further endocrinological diseases.

CASE 12: RECURRENT HYPOGLYCAEMIA IN A YOUNG WOMAN WITH TYPE 1 DIABETES

Vincent McAulay and Brian M Frier

History

A 29-year-old female accountant who developed type 1 diabetes in 1985 rapidly achieved excellent glycaemic control on twice-daily human Mixtard 30 insulin (NovoNordisk), which contains 30% soluble and 70% isophane insulin (0.34 U/kg/day). For several years she maintained strict glycaemic control; HbA1c values were at the upper end of the non-diabetic range. Preprandial blood glucose was usually around 4–5 mmol/L and lower values were seldom recorded.

She followed a healthy diet and was physically active, exercising several times a week. At routine review in February 1996 she reported recurrent episodes of hypoglycaemia, none of which had been severe. At that time, her HbA1c was 5.4% (non-diabetic range 5–6.5%), her insulin dose remained at 0.34 U/kg day and she was advised to relax her glycaemic control. However, when reviewed 6 months later, the HbA1c was unchanged and she had recorded frequent asymptomatic biochemical hypoglycaemia. She admitted to having increased her total insulin dose to maintain her preprandial blood glucose in the normal range (4–5 mmol/L). Soon afterwards she experienced an episode of severe hypoglycaemia that was treated with intramuscular glucagon.

In 1998, nocturnal hypoglycaemia was a recurring problem, and on one occasion she suffered a convulsion. Her daytime symptoms of hypoglycaemia had diminished in intensity and she often documented blood glucose concentrations of around 2.0 mmol/L with no associated warning symptoms. A basal-bolus regimen was commenced with insulin lispro (Humalog; Eli Lilly) before meals and isophane insulin (Humulin I; Eli Lilly) at bedtime. Despite advice to the contrary, she continued to maintain strict glycaemic control and had three further episodes of severe hypoglycaemia during the subsequent year. When she awoke from sleep one morning, she was unable to move her left arm and leg for 2 hours. This transient hemiplegia was associated with severe hypoglycaemia. She finally agreed to relax her glycaemic control, and reduced her total insulin dose.

Commentary

Strict glycaemic control delays the onset and slows the progression of microvascular complications in type 1 diabetes but is associated with a higher frequency of severe hypoglycaemia and significant morbidity.[1,2] Neuroglycopenia causes a rapid deterioration in cerebral function, and severe hypoglycaemia can provoke convulsions, coma, physical injury and neurological syndromes such as transient hemiparesis (Box 1). Hypoglycaemia of any severity is disabling and can disrupt all aspects of everyday life.

Box 1   Neurological and psychological manifestations of severe hypoglycaemia

Neurological
- Focal or generalized convulsions
- Coma
- Hemiparesis, transient ischaemic attacks
- Ataxia, choreoathetosis
- Focal neurological deficits
- Decortication

Psychological
- Cognitive impairment
- Behavioural/personality and mood changes
- Aggressive behaviour, automatism, psychosis

The blood glucose levels at which physiological responses to hypoglycaemia are triggered (glycaemic thresholds) are not fixed, but can be influenced by preceding glycaemic exposure. In type 1 diabetes the thresholds are modified by *strict* glycaemic control (HbA1c within or near the non-diabetic range[3]) and by episodic or *antecedent* hypoglycaemia.[4,5] Exposure to antecedent hypoglycaemia for 60 minutes or more diminishes the magnitude of neuroendocrine and symptomatic responses to subsequent episodes of hypoglycaemia occurring within the following 24–48 hours.[5] The thresholds for the onset of symptoms and the secretion of counter-regulatory hormones are affected so that a more profound hypoglycaemic stimulus is required to trigger these responses. During periods of strict glycaemic control the cerebral uptake of glucose is maintained during hypoglycaemia, so preserving cognitive function despite a low blood glucose.[6] This is a manifestation of cerebral adaptation to prolonged exposure to neuroglycopenia, but it is maladaptive as the early symptomatic warning of hypoglycaemia is absent, risking progression to severe neuroglycopenia.

These effects on perception of symptoms of hypoglycaemia may lead to the acquired syndrome of impaired awareness of hypoglycaemia (as had occurred in the present case). This acquired syndrome affects 25% of people with type 1 diabetes,[5,7] is more common with increasing duration of diabetes,[8] has a sixfold higher rate of severe hypoglycaemia than those with normal awareness,[9] and co-segregates with counter-regulatory deficiencies[10] which are also common in type 1 diabetes of long duration. When strict glycaemic control is induced with intensive insulin therapy in individuals with counter-regulatory deficiencies, the frequency of severe hypoglycaemia is greatly increased.[11]

Most insulin regimens cause nocturnal hyperinsulinaemia and predispose to nocturnal hypoglycaemia, which occurs in up to 50% of people treated with insulin, is asymptomatic in 25–75% of episodes and may last for up to 6 hours.[12] Clinical features of nocturnal hypoglycaemia include morning headaches, nightmares and poor quality of sleep, and suspicion of a nocturnal fall in blood glucose should be verified by biochemical testing. Hypoglycaemia during sleep is associated with varying morbidity, and occasional fatalities (the 'dead in bed syndrome').[13] Nocturnal hypoglycaemia may induce impaired awareness of hypoglycaemia through the pathogenetic mechanism of antecedent hypoglycaemia.[14,15]

What did I learn from this case?

Strict glycaemic control, although desirable to protect against the development of vascular complications, has potential risks. These include modification of the symptomatic response to hypoglycaemia to induce impaired awareness, and to attenuate counter-regulation. Intensive insulin therapy may therefore increase the risk of severe hypoglycaemia and potentially serious neurological consequences such as convulsions or transient hemiplegia. The insulin regimen should be tailored to the daily requirements of the individual so that the risk of severe hypoglycaemia is minimized. In the DCCT, only 5% of participants were able to maintain their HbA1c within the non-diabetic range,[16,17] but this target may be undesirable as it predisposes to impaired awareness of hypoglycaemia and counter-regulatory deficiencies.[3]

How much did this case alter my approach to the care and treatment of my patients with diabetes?

Fixed mixtures of insulin often cause unwanted nocturnal hyperinsulinaemia, predisposing to unrecognized hypoglycaemia. When isophane insulin is administered before the evening meal, nocturnal hypoglycaemia often occurs at around 3.00–4.00 am,[18] while soluble insulin before a late evening meal can cause hypoglycaemia in the early hours of the night.[19] To avoid nocturnal hypoglycaemia useful therapeutic manoeuvres include the use of a fast-acting insulin analogue before the evening meal or the evening dose of isophane insulin can be deferred until bedtime.

Some patients have a compulsion to maintain strict glycaemic control, are obsessional about frequent blood glucose monitoring and try to maintain their blood glucose within a near-normal range. When this causes serious problems with hypoglycaemia they must be persuaded to reduce their total insulin dose and relax their glycaemic control.

References

1. The Diabetes Control and Complications Trial Research Group. Epidemiology of severe hypoglycemia in the Diabetes Control and Complications Trial. *Am J Med* 1991; 90: 450–9.

2. Reichard P, Rosenqvist U, Britz A. Intensified conventional insulin treatment and neuropsychological impairment. *BMJ* 1991; 303: 1439–42.

3. Kinsley BT, Widom B, Simonson DC. Differential regulation of counterregulatory hormone secretion and symptoms during hypoglycemia in IDDM. *Diabetes Care* 1995; 18: 17–26.

4. Bolli G. Prevention and treatment of hypoglycaemia unawareness in type 1 diabetes mellitus. *Acta Diabetol* 1998; 35: 183–93.

5. Frier BM, Fisher BM. Impaired hypoglycaemia awareness. In: Frier BM, Fisher BM, eds. *Hypoglycaemia in Clinical Diabetes*. Chichester: John Wiley & Sons, 1999: 111–46.

6. Boyle PJ, Kempers SF, O'Connor AM, Nagy RJ. Brain glucose uptake and unawareness of hypoglycemia in patients with insulin-dependent diabetes mellitus. *N Engl J Med* 1995; 333: 1726–31.

7. Gerich JE, Mokan M, Veneman T, Korytkowski M, Mitrakou M. Hypoglycemia unawareness. *Endocr Rev* 1991; 12: 356–71.

8. Pramming S, Thorsteinsson B, Bendston I, Binder C. Symptomatic hypoglycaemia in 411 Type 1 diabetic patients. *Diabetic Med* 1991; 8: 217–22.

9. Gold AE, MacLeod KM, Frier BM. Frequency of severe hypoglycemia in patients with type 1 diabetes with impaired awareness of hypoglycemia. *Diabetes Care* 1994; 17: 697–703.

10. Ryder REJ, Owens DR, Hayes DM, Ghatei MA, Bloom SR. Unawareness of hypoglycaemia and inadequate hypoglycaemic counterregulation: no causal relation with diabetic autonomic neuropathy. *BMJ* 1990; 301: 783–7.

11. White NH, Skor DA, Cryer PE, Levandoski LA, Bier DM, Santiago JV. Identification of type 1 diabetic patients at increased risk for hypoglycemia during intensive insulin therapy. *N Engl J Med* 1983; **308**: 485 91.

12. Tattersall RB. Frequency, causes and treatment of hypoglycaemia. In: Frier BM, Fisher BM eds. *Hypoglycaemia in Clinical Diabetes*. Chichester: John Wiley & Sons, 1999: 55–87.

13. Fisher BM and Heller SR. Mortality, cardiovascular morbidity and possible effects of hypoglycaemia on diabetic complications, In: Frier BM, Fisher BM eds. *Hypoglycaemia in Clinical Diabetes*. Chichester: John Wiley & Sons, 1999: 167–86.

14. Veneman T, Mitrakou A, Mokan M, Cryer P, Gerich J. Induction of hypoglycemia unawareness by asymptomatic nocturnal hypoglycemia. *Diabetes* 1993; **42**: 1233–7.

15. Fanelli CG, Paramore DS, Hershey T et al. Impact of nocturnal hypoglycemia on hypoglycaemic cognitive dysfunction in type 1 diabetes. *Diabetes* 1998; **47**: 1920–7.

16. The Diabetes Control and Complications Trial Research Group. The effects of intensive insulin treatment of diabetes on the development and progression of long-term complications in insulin-dependent diabetes mellitus. *N Engl J Med* 1993; **329**: 977–86.

17. The Diabetes Control and Complications Trial Research Group. Implementation of treatment protocols in the Diabetes Control and Complications Trial. *Diabetes Care* 1995; **18**: 361–76.

18. Pramming S, Thorsteinsson B, Bendtson I, Ronn B, Binder C. Nocturnal hypoglycaemia in patients receiving conventional treatment with insulin. *BMJ* 1985; **291**: 376–9.

19. Vervoort G, Goldschmidt HMG, van Doorn LG. Nocturnal blood glucose profiles in patients with type 1 diabetes mellitus on multiple (> 4) daily insulin injection regimens. *Diab Med* 1996; **13**: 794–9.

Case 13: Frequent hypoglycaemia in a boy with type 1 diabetes

Peter GF Swift

History

Kevin developed type 1 diabetes at 15 months of age. He was not dehydrated nor acidotic at that time and was managed entirely out of hospital.

His metabolic control in the early years was satisfactory, with twice-daily injections of a mixture of soluble (Actrapid) and NPH (Insulatard) insulins at a dose of about 0.7 units/kg/day.

His mother had trained as a nurse and his father was a hospital-based electronics engineer. They became involved in the organization of the local Parents Branch of the British Diabetic Association (now Diabetes (UK)). Kevin's mother had been taught to estimate carbohydrate portions, and dietary assessments suggested that she had developed a rather rigid approach to dietary intake.

By the age of 9 or 10 years, as he became more independent at home and at school, Kevin's glycaemic control became less satisfactory with an HbA1c around 8.5%. Just before his 11th birthday he began to experience frequent hypoglycaemic episodes, particularly in the evening, after school. His mother reduced his evening insulin. Over the next few weeks the hypoglycaemias began to occur at school so that his emergency supplies of biscuits and chocolate in the school were rapidly exhausted. His morning insulin was reduced and the mother changed to fresh bottles of insulin in case of an error of formulation.

Because the hypoglycaemic episodes were becoming more frequent and severe, despite the reduced insulin dose, the diabetes specialist nurse was consulted and she advised a further reduction in dosage.

Shortly after this, Kevin attended the diabetic clinic. All his recorded blood glucose measurements were within or below the normal range and his HbA1c had fallen to 5.3% (NR 4–6.1%). He seemed well in himself, although there was now some anxiety because the hypoglycaemic attacks were affecting his schoolwork and some were also occurring at night. On several occasions he had woken his parents at 2 or 3 am with a piercing scream and they had found him semi-conscious, sweating profusely and with jerking movements of his limbs. They had been able to reverse the severe hypoglycaemia with Hypostop® and chocolate biscuits on two occasions but he had needed glucagon on another occasion. By this stage he was taking minimal doses of insulin and the parents were asking if something else was wrong or whether his pancreas had started to work again. There were no symptoms or signs of other conditions such as thyroid dysfunction, Addison's disease or coeliac disease.

Treatment and outcome

It was suggested that if frequent hypoglycaemias continued to occur, the insulin injections might be discontinued, and that measurements should be made of fasting C-peptide, cortisol, thyroid function and antibodies against the adrenal, thyroid, gluten/endomysium and perhaps the islet cells.

The father called the consultant a few days later to report that further severe hypoglycaemias had occurred on tiny doses of insulin and his wife had now stopped the insulin.

The consultant asked whether the parents personally supervised every injection. They were confident that they saw Kevin give nearly all the injections. When the consultant advised that the parents checked every source of insulin in case Kevin had been injecting extra insulin to cause hypoglycaemia, they expressed considerable disbelief and some anger. They could not imagine that their otherwise well-behaved, generally cooperative 10-year-old could possibly be so devious. Nevertheless the parents agreed to check out and collect all the insulin bottles and syringes. The evening injection was missed out as planned and also the next morning dose. Kevin was due to go swimming with his father that morning. He became agitated and only reluctantly went to the swimming pool, where his blood glucose was measured and was > 25 mmol/L for the first time in several weeks.

Back at home the story became clear. Kevin had always had a very sweet tooth. He desperately wanted more chocolates so he thought the way to do that without his parents knowing was to eat whatever sweets and chocolate he could and to control these binges with extra doses of Actrapid stolen from the fridge. This seemed to work so he decided to inject more and eat more. Most young people dislike hypoglycaemias (see Figure 1) but he admitted feeling a sort of 'high' as his blood sugar dropped and as he ate more chocolate to combat the hypo. However, he began to lose control of this because the hypos became more severe and occurred at different times of the day and the night. Obviously, his parents did not suspect that he might be injecting excessive doses of insulin so he had to keep up the pretence until his apparent insulin dose was reduced to nothing. 'I tried to control it myself but then it took control of me'.

Management was as follows:

1. The story was explained carefully to Kevin and his parents without any criticism or judgement.
2. Kevin's extraordinarily clever reasoning and actions were acknowledged but the stealing, secrecy and deceit were deemed unacceptable.

this is me fieling funny
its not rerey nise but
they give me sum choclat

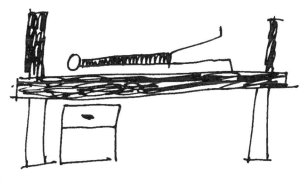

Figure 1 *'What I don't like about diabetes' by child aged 8 years, Diabetic camp 1996.*

3. We agreed to more flexibility in the diet and encouraged more trust and cooperation between Kevin and his parents.
4. The use of one of the newer rapid-acting analogue insulins was suggested for episodes of hyperglycaemia, or before bigger meals, or occasions when Kevin might want to eat special treats. It was thought that this type of insulin might cause fewer hypoglycaemic reactions.

Kevin's overall glycaemic control has not been satisfactory, with HbA1c = 8.7%, but he has not experienced any major hypoglycaemias nor any serious adverse psychological effects. He has learnt to treat hyperglycaemia with additional doses of rapid-acting insulin.

Learning points

1. No age is exempt from factitious hypoglycaemia (or DKA from insulin omission).

2. If insulin doses drop severely and unexpectedly, factitious insulin overdosing must be considered, although Addison's disease and coeliac disease should be excluded.

3. Despite a child's deception he or she must make something positive out of the situation. The child must be given unconditional support and be able to move forward into a position of greater trust and understanding because diabetes is a diabolically difficult disease with many confusing and conflicting emotions, especially in the very young.

4. If the problems extend to other areas of misbehaviour, then an expert psychologist or child psychiatrist may be required.

Further reading

O'Brien IAD, Lewin IG, Frier BM, Rodman H, Genuth S, Corrall RJM. Factitious diabetic instability. *Diab Med* 1985; 2: 392–4.

Orr DP, Eccles T, Lawlor R, Golden M. Surreptitious insulin administration in adolescents with insulin-dependent diabetes mellitus. *JAMA* 1986; 256: 3227–30.

Swift PGF. Hypoglycaemia in children with diabetes. In: Frier BM, Fisher BM, eds. *Hypoglycaemia in Clinical Diabetes*. Chichester: Wiley & Sons, 1999: 219.

CASE 14: TYPE 1 OR TYPE 2 DIABETES?

Ulrich Julius

History

Patient GR was born on 09/10/76. His grandmother suffers from diabetes mellitus which is very well compensated. The patient had no relevant history up to March 1998 when he had a torsion fracture of his left ankle joint. Four weeks later the screws were due to be removed, but preoperatively an elevated blood glucose concentration (29.5 mmol/L) was detected. The patient was transferred to another hospital where he was put on insulin treatment. He injected a dose of regular insulin (8 IU Actrapid) three times daily and NPH insulin (12/0/0/8 IU protaphan) in the morning and at night. In the following months the insulin dosage had to be decreased because of rather low blood glucose concentrations. Finally, only 4 IU protaphan were injected at night. In January 1999 the insulin therapy was stopped. In June 1999 the HbA1 level was 10.9%, and the blood glucose level was 4.9 mmol/L. Autoantibodies against islet cells (ICA) were found, as well as autoantibodies against insulin. At that time the blood cell count and major laboratory findings (transaminases, gamma-glutamyltransferase, alkaline phosphatase, bilirubin, lipase, amylase, creatinine, uric acid, triglycerides, serum cholesterol, HDL cholesterol) were in the normal range. In July 1999 the HbA1c level was 6.6% and the blood glucose concentration was 5.64 mmol/L. In August 1999 an examination by the ophthalmologist did not reveal any diabetic retinopathy. At the end of August 1999, the HbA1c level was 8.1% and the postprandial serum glucose level was 13.58 mmol/L. His body weight was 70.0 kg, his height was 1.69 m. We performed a glucagon test (injecting 1 mg glucagon intravenously) and measured the parameters shown in Table 1.

The normal range for insulin is 0.06–0.25 nmol/L; thus the basal insulin level of the patient was seen to be increased. The basal C-peptide level was in the

Table 1 Blood glucose, insulin and C-peptide levels before and 6 min after intravenous glucagon

Time of sampling	Blood glucose (mmol/L)	Insulin (nmol/L)	C-peptide (nmol/L)
0 min	12.27	0.32	0.81
6 min	13.86	0.33	1.32

normal range (0.33–1.07 nmol/L). After glucagon, the insulin level was not increased as expected, but the C-peptide level rose. As this post-glucagon C-peptide level exceeded the normal limit of 1.1 nmol/L, one could suspect that our patient suffered from a type 2 diabetes mellitus. Moreover, the fasting proinsulin concentration was clearly elevated (11.2 pmol/L; normal range 0.7–4.3 pmol/L). No autoantibodies were detected against islet cells (ICA), against glutamate decarboxylase II or against islet cell antigen 2, but autoantibodies against insulin were found.

In August 1999 we suggested that the patient measure his pre- and post-prandial (1.5 hours after the main meals) blood glucose levels on a regular basis. The results of this self-monitoring are shown in Table 2.

Table 2 Self-monitoring of blood glucose pre- (first line) and post-prandially (second line) in August 1999

Date	Morning	Lunchtime	Dinnertime	At night
14/08/99	5.3	5.8	5.1	5.9
	12.0	10.1	11.8	
15/08/99	5.0	5.6	5.2	5.8
	12.0	12.1	11.7	
18/08/99	4.9	5.1	4.8	5.7
	11.0	11.5	10.0	

As postprandial blood glucose concentrations were increased, we started an acarbose treatment (three $\times$ 50 mg Glucobay). We avoided insulin treatment at that time because the patient was a member of the police force.

In October 1999, the blood glucose levels shown in Table 3 were documented by the patient. Thus, acarbose did improve the postprandial glycaemic control. The HbA1c level at that time was 7.9%.

Table 3 Self-monitoring of blood glucose pre- (first line) and post-prandially (second line) in October 1999

Date	Morning	Lunchtime	Dinnertime	At night
01/10/99	5.0	4.8	5.1	5.9
	9.0	8.8	8.9	
09/10/99	5.2	5.3	4.9	6.0
	9.4	9.1	9.0	
17/10/99	5.1	5.2	4.7	5.8
	9.0	9.1	8.9	

However, in the following months, a deterioration of the blood glucose levels took place (Table 4). The HbA1c level on 12/01/00 was 11.9%, the blood glucose level was 12.99 mmol/L. We stopped the acarbose treatment and started repaglinide (3 × 0.5 mg Novonorm). In the following days, postprandial blood glucose concentrations exceeded 10.0 mmol/L. Therefore the patient was switched to an insulin therapy again: (8/6/6 IU lispro insulin before the main meals). This brought postprandial blood glucose values to about 8.0 mmol/L.

Table 4   Self-monitoring of blood glucose pre- (first line) and post-prandially (second line)in December 1999/January 2000

Date	Morning	Lunchtime	Dinnertime	At night
16/12/99	6.0	6.1	5.9	6.0
	12.0	10.1	9.8	
24/12/99	6.0	6.2	5.8	6.0
	11.0	10.1	9.9	
02/01/00	5.9	5.1	6.5	6.0
	10.0	14.1	10.1	

In July 2000 the postprandial blood glucose concentration as measured by the laboratory was 7.57 mmol/L, but the HbA1c level was 9.3%. The blood cell count, thyroid hormones and lipid concentrations were in the normal range. In the following months, preprandial glucose concentrations as measured by the patient himself were about 5.8 mmol/L. Postprandial blood glucose levels rose up to 9 mmol/L. We checked the glycaemic control of the patient in early November again and observed an HbA1c level of 10.3%; the blood glucose as measured in the laboratory was 15.04 mmol/L. We checked thoroughly to find out whether the patient/measured his blood glucose values correctly and could not find any irregularity. The preprandial glucose concentrations as measured by the patient remained between 4.8 and 6.5 mmol/L; however, postprandial values exceeded 10 mmol/L but were below 12 mmol/L. At night, the patient documented blood glucose levels between 6.0 and 7.1 mmol/L. We added acarbose again (3 × 50 mg Glucobay), the postprandial blood glucose concentrations improved. In November 2000 we also rechecked the level of autoantibodies and this time we detected autoantibodies against glutamate decarboxylase II and against insulin.

What did we learn from this case?

Evidently, the patient has a type 1 diabetes mellitus. This was proved by the positive autoantibody findings. On the other hand, he still exhibited a sufficient C-peptide response to glucagon, meaning that his secretory capacity for insulin was not diminished. During the initial insulin therapy, hypoglycaemic episodes were occurring, which led the treating physician to finally stop the insulin injections. It appeared that the patient had postprandial glucose elevations leading to an increased HbA1c level. His pre-meal glucose concentrations were in the optimal range. We started with an acarbose treatment in order to lower the postprandial rise of glucose. Indeed, we were successful in this respect, although the HbA1c level did not reach the optimal range. In the following months, the glycaemic control deteriorated, especially postprandially. For some days, we administered repaglinide and then decided to start a prandial insulin injection scheme. We administered rather low doses of a short-acting insulin. In this way, postprandial glucose elevations could be diminished again. As postprandial glucose concentrations exceeded 10 mmol/L we eventually added acarbose to the insulin regime again.

Case 15: From Hyperinsulinaemia in Childhood to Diabetes in Adulthood

Markku Laakso and Hanna Huopio

History

A 41-year-old Finnish woman had a history of hypoglycaemic episodes when she was less than 2 years old. She had weakness, headache, nausea, tremor and even unconsciousness during fasting, which disappeared very quickly after eating. Her mother had diabetes. At the age of 6 years the patient was diagnosed with grand mal epilepsy at the university hospital, and has been on anticonvulsive medication ever since. During her two pregnancies the patient developed gestational diabetes and was treated with short-acting insulin. Glucose tolerance normalized after the delivery.

The patient's second child, a girl, developed severe hypoglycaemia immediately after birth. Despite maximal feeding and intravenous glucose administration (15–20 mg/kg/min), she had persistent hypoglycaemia (about 2 mmol/L). During hypoglycaemia (blood glucose level was 2.4 mmol/L) the simultaneously measured insulin level was as high as 164 mU/L, indicating severe hyperinsulinaemia. Her macrosomic appearance at birth (birth weight was 5.36 kg) reflected fetal hyperinsulinaemia. Because of persistent non-ketotic hyperinsulinaemic hypoglycaemia, the baby was diagnosed as having congenital hyperinsulinaemia (CHI; also known as PPHI, persistent hyperinsulinaemic hypoglycaemia of infancy). Diazoxide therapy proved to be effective in her case and normalized the blood glucose levels. At the age of 10 years she is still on low-dose diazoxide therapy (3 mg/kg/day divided into three doses). DNA testing revealed that she had a heterozygous GAG-AAG substitution in codon 1506 of the sulfonylurea receptor-1 gene (*SUR1*), which results in an amino acid change from glutamic acid to lysine (E1506K).

Examination and investigations

The patient was invited to undergo metabolic studies carried out at the Department of Medicine, University of Kuopio. Genetic testing showed that, like her baby daughter, she also had the heterozygous SUR1-E1506K mutation. At the time of these metabolic studies, she was 41 years old, her height was 165.5 cm, her weight 68 kg (body mass index 24.8 kg/m²), and her blood pressure levels were 106/70 mmHg. Her total cholesterol was 5.1 mmol/L, low-density lipoprotein cholesterol 3.3 mmol/L, high-density lipoprotein cholesterol 1.5 mmol/L and total triglycerides 1.3 mmol/L. Her glycated haemoglobin A1c was 6.0% (normal range 4–6%), fasting blood glucose 6.2 mmol/L, 1-hour glucose 13.3 mmol/L and 2-hour glucose 13.1 mmol/L in an oral glucose tolerance test (75 g of glucose), fulfilling the criteria for diabetes. The corresponding insulin concentrations were 6.0, 13.2 and 10.5 mU/L, and C-peptide levels were 0.49, 0.90 and 0.93 nmol/L respectively, indicating that she had low post-challenge insulin and C-peptide levels. In the euglycaemic hyperinsulinaemic clamp (insulin infusion rate of 80 mU/kg/min; blood glucose during the clamp 5.0 mmol/L) her M-value (glucose infusion rate) was 13.8 mg/min/kg, indicating that her insulin sensitivity was completely normal (mean for the control group was 10.1 mg/min/kg). In contrast, insulin area during the first 10 minutes of an intravenous glucose tolerance test was 25.25 mU/L/min, suggesting that her first-phase insulin secretion was only about 4% of the normal value (mean of controls 571 mU/L/min).

Commentary

Our patient had an unusual history of abnormalities in glucose metabolism. She had episodes of hypoglycaemia in early childhood, gestational diabetes during both pregnancies, and finally diabetes due to a clear insulin secretion deficiency. The patient's diabetes is well controlled with diet only, and she does not have any long-term complications of diabetes.

Our patient, and her daughter, were heterozygous for the E1506K mutation of the *SUR1* gene. Electrophysiological studies showed that the SUR1-E1506K mutation leads to a reduction, but not a complete loss, of ATP-sensitive potassium (K_{ATP}) channels. The mutant channels are insensitive to metabolic inhibition but are activated by diazoxide.[1] The patient had hypoglycaemic symptoms during her childhood but was never diagnosed as having CHI. In contrast, the patient's daughter had severe symptoms after her birth and was diagnosed as having CHI.

CHI is a rare genetic disorder characterized by a dysregulation of insulin secretion that leads to recurrent or persistent hypoglycaemia. Mutations in four different genes have been associated with CHI.[2–5] Most mutations are associated with the beta-cell K_{ATP} channel, which plays a major role in the regulation of insulin secretion. The K_{ATP} channel consists of two types of protein subunits: SUR1 and the inward rectifying potassium channel Kir 6.2. Mutations in the *SUR1* gene are the major known cause for CHI,[2] but a few mutations in Kir6.2 have also been reported.[3] Most of these mutations are inherited recessively. A gain-of-function mutation in the glucokinase gene causes a dominant form of CHI.[4] Furthermore, mutations in the glutamate dehydrogenase gene can cause CHI with hyperammonaemia.[5]

The patient and her daughter belonged to a large Finnish pedigree carrying the SUR1 mutation E1506K.[1] Altogether seven paediatric patients diagnosed with CHI carried that mutation. Five of them presented with hypoglycaemia during the first few hours after birth. In the other two cases, the symptoms appeared at the age of 5 and 7 months. Four of five patients who were treated with diazoxide had a good response. At least two of the mothers had had symptoms that could be classified as hypoglycaemia during the first 2 years of life, although low blood glucose was not documented. All except one of the mothers had gestational diabetes (including our patient).

Type 2 diabetes is a heterogeneous disorder that results from varying degrees of abnormalities in insulin secretion and insulin action.[6] The genetic background of this disease is known only in a minority of subtypes such as monogenic maturity-onset diabetes of the young (MODY),[7] a disorder characterized by deficient insulin secretion.

Our patient with the SUR1-E1506K mutation, like most CHI patients, probably had a slow progressive loss of beta-cell function.[8] The mechanism for impaired insulin secretion could be due to beta-cell apoptosis.[9] Supporting this notion is a transgenic mouse model of CHI overexpressing a dominant negative form of Kir6.2 in pancreatic beta cells. In these mice hyperinsulinaemia is evident in the neonatal period but insulin deficiency, attributed to apoptosis, develops later.[10] The association of mutations in the *SUR1* gene with type 2 diabetes has remained unclear. Some studies,[11,12] but not all,[13] have found an association of variants in the *SUR1* gene and type 2 diabetes. We did not find the SUR1-E1506K mutation in 80 adult type 2 diabetic patients.

Insulin resistance in peripheral tissues is a characteristic finding in patients with type 2 diabetes. The pancreas compensates for insulin resistance by secreting more insulin to overcome impaired insulin action in peripheral tissues. When the pancreas fails to secrete enough insulin, hyperglycaemia develops. Our case does not follow this generally accepted paradigm. The primary defect in glucose metabolism was an inherited dysregulation of insulin secretion in the presence of completely normal insulin sensitivity. In fact, our patient was able to compensate for her severe defect in insulin secretion by high insulin sensitivity. At the time of diagnosis of diabetes she was able to lose weight, which almost normalized glucose metabolism. Our case demonstrates that lifestyle changes leading to an improvement in insulin sensitivity are not only effective in the prevention of diabetes, but can effectively compensate for impaired insulin secretion and maintain normal glucose tolerance in diabetic patients.

References

1. Huopio H, Reimann F, Ashfield R et al. Dominantly inherited hyperinsulism caused by a mutation in the sulfonylurea receptor type 1. *J Clin Invest* 2000; 106: 897–906.

2. Thomas PM, Cote GJ, Wohllk N et al. Mutations in the sulfonylurea receptor gene in familial persistent hyperinsulinemic hypoglycemia of infancy. *Science* 1995; **268**: 426–9.

3. Thomas P, Ye Y, Lightner E. Mutations of the pancreatic islet inward rectifier Kir6.2 also leads to familial persistent hyperinsulinemic hypoglycemia of infancy. *Hum Mol Genet* 1996; **5**: 1809–12.

4. Glaser B, Kesavan P, Heyman M et al. Familial hyperinsulinism caused by an activating glucokinase mutation. *N Engl J Med* 1998; **338**: 226–30.

5. Stanley CA, Lieu YK, Hsu BY et al. Hyperinsulism and hyperammonemia in infants with regulatory mutations of the glutamate dehydrogenase gene. *N Engl J Med* 1998; **338**: 1352–7.

6. DeFronzo RA, Bonadonna RC, Ferrannini E. Pathogenesis of NIDDM. A balanced overview. *Diabetes Care* 1992; **15**: 318–68.

7. Doria A, Plengvidhya N. Recent advances in the genetics of maturity-onset diabetes of the young and other forms of autosomal dominant diabetes. *Curr Opin Endocrinol Diabetes* 2000; **7**: 203–10.

8. Leibowitz G, Glaser B, Higazi AA, Salameh M, Cerasi E, Landau H. Hyper-insulinemic hyperglycemia of infancy (nesidioblastosis) in clinical remission: high incidence of diabetes mellitus and persistent beta-cell dysfunction at long-term follow-up. *J Clin Endocrinol Metab* 1995; **80**: 386–92.

9. Kassem SA, Ariel I, Thornton PS, Scheimberg I, Glaser B. Beta-cell proliferation and apoptosis in the developing normal human pancreas and in hyperinsulism of infancy. *Diabetes* 2000; **49**: 1325–33.

10. Miki T, Tashiro F, Iwanaga T et al. Abnormalities of pancreatic islets by targeted expression of a dominant-negative K_{ATP} channel. *Proc Natl Acad Sci USA* 1997; **94**: 11969–73.

11. Inoue H, Ferrer J, Welling CM et al. Sequence variants in the sulfonylurea receptor (SUR) gene are associated with NIDDM in Caucasians. *Diabetes* 1996; **45**: 825–31.

12. t'Hart LM, de Knijff P, Dekker JM et al. Variants in the sulfonylurea receptor gene: association of the exon 16-3t variant with Type II diabetes mellitus in Dutch Caucasians. *Diabetologia* 1999; **42**: 617–20.

13. Ishiyama-Shigenoto S, Yamada K, Yuan X et al. Clinical characterization of polymorphisms in the sulphonylurea receptor 1 gene in Japanese subjects with type 2 diabetes mellitus. *Diabetic Med* 1998; **15**: 826–9.

CASE 16: SEVERE OBESITY AND DIABETES IN YOUTH

Gabriele Riccardi, Olga Vaccaro

History

A 24-year-old man was admitted to hospital because of persistent, marked hyperglycaemia and severe obesity. Both parents were alive and free from either diabetes or obesity, as was his only brother. He was born after a full-term uncomplicated pregnancy; during the neonatal period diffuse muscular hypotonia was noted. In infancy motor development was delayed and the child was incapable of independent walking until the age of 3. By age 8 the child had become obese and at age 18 he weighed 103 kg. Delayed development of secondary sexual characters at adolescence led to the diagnosis of hypogonadism and chronic treatment with testosterone. Five years before admission, at age 19, the patient had received a diagnosis of type 2 diabetes mellitus manifesting with polyuria, polydipsia, urinary tract infection and hyperglycaemia (220 mg/dL). Fasting and stimulated C peptide plasma concentrations at the time of diagnosis were 3.3 and 7.0 ng/mL, respectively. A low calory diet was prescribed, but the patient was incapable of complying. Glucose control deteriorated progressively, leading to the prescription of metformin, which the patient took regularly thereafter at a dosage of 2500 mg/day. Because of poor glucose control after a few months insulin was also prescribed. Glucose control had always been poor and had deteriorated further in the last few months. Several days before admission dysuria had developed.

On admission the patient was slightly dehydrated, his temperature was 36.4°C, pulse was 100 beats/min, blood pressure 130/70 mmHg, plasma glucose 490 mg/dL, glycated haemoglobin 14% and plasma tryglycerides 400 mg/dL. The urine was positive for glucose and negative for ketone bodies, the sediment contained white cells and bacteria. Other blood chemicals, enzymes and haematological values were normal. Physical examination revealed marked obesity (BMI 43 kg/m^2) with a central distribution of body fat, short stature, short hands and feet, characteristic facial features (a narrow bifrontral diameter, almond-shaped eyes and down-turned corners of the mouth). Hypogonadism was also present and he was mentally retarded.

Type 2 diabetes is a common disease and its prevalence is particularly high in obese individuals. However, when the diagnosis is made at a young age, other, less common types of diabetes must be excluded before the diagnosis of type 2 diabetes is firmly established. In this particular patient the difficulties in achieving blood glucose control, the coexistence of morbid obesity manifesting early in life and the impossibility of controlling progressive weight increase and hyperglycaemia further stress the need for re-evaluation of the diagnosis and treatment strategies.

Type 1 diabetes can be excluded on the basis of clinical criteria (no history of ketoacidosis, long-term history of non-insulin requirement). The absence of markers of autoimmunity (anti-glutamic acid decarboxylase antibody, insulin autoantibodies) further supported exclusion of type 1 diabetes.

The described clinical and immunological characteristics combined with onset at age < 25 years pose the differential diagnosis with maturity-onset diabetes of the young (MODY), a type of diabetes associated with genetic defects of B-cell function and autosomal dominant inheritance.[1] However, neither diabetes nor hyperglycaemia could be detected in the parents and their first-degree relatives, thus making MODY highly unlikely.[2] Endocrinopathies associated with diabetes (i.e. Cushing's syndrome, hyperthyroidism, acromegaly) were ruled out on clinical grounds and biochemical measurements: urine free cortisol was 207 nmol/dL, and plasma ACTH 4.8 pmol/L, TSH 2.7 mU/L, GH 0.5 µg/L.

The concomitant severe obesity starting at a young age suggested the hypothesis of a genetically related syndrome of obesity and diabetes. Early-onset morbid obesity is a cardinal feature of Prader–Willi syndrome (PWS)[3] and is often complicated with diabetes. PWS is a rare (one per 10,000–15,000 live births) autosomal dominant disorder involving the long arm of chromosome 15. It is caused more frequently by a deletion of the paternal chromosome, or more rarely by maternal uniparental disomy 15 or an imprinting mutation resulting in the maternal imprinting pattern. The syndrome tends to be overdiagnosed in infancy and underdiagnosed in adults, the development of a comprehensive clinical diagnostic scoring system (see Box 26.1) has greatly reduced the need for unnecessary laborious molecular diagnostic investigations.[3,4] Our patient met seven out of eight major diagnostic criteria for PWS (criteria 2–8 in Box 1) including deletion of the long arm of chromosome 15 q11–13. Minor criteria 2, 4, 6 and 10 were also met, thus giving a total score of 9 and allowing diagnosis.

Treatment and outcome

Hyperglycaemia is frequent in PWS, although the mechanisms are not fully understood. Insulin resistance has been documented in diabetes complicating PWS, as well as a reduced insulin production.[5] Insulin-dependent and rapidly progressive microvascular complications, although rare, have also been described in association with PWS, thus stressing the need for careful monitoring of diabetic complications in these patients.[6] Glucose control in PWS is very difficult,

---

Box 1 Summary of diagnostic criteria for Prader–Willi syndrome

Major criteria
1) Feeding problems in infancy
2) Neonatal and infantile central hypotonia
3) Excessive or rapid weight gain before 6 years of age
4) Characteristic facial features
5) Hypogonadism
6) Global developmental delay before 6 years of age
7) Hyperphagia/obsession with food
8) Deletion 5 q11–13 or other cytogenetic abnormalities of the PW chromosome region

Minor criteria
1) Decreased fetal movement or infantile lethargy
2) Characteristic behaviour problems
3) Sleep disturbances or sleep apnoea
4) Short stature for genetic background
5) Hypopigmentation
6) Small hands and/or feet
7) Narrow hands with straight ulnar border
8) Eye abnormalities (esotropia, myopia)
9) Thick viscous saliva
10) Speech articulation defects
11) Skin picking

Major criteria score 1, minor criteria score 0.5; a total score of 8 is necessary for diagnosis. Major criteria must comprise at least 5 points of the total score.

---

as the syndrome includes pathologic hyperphagia, obsession with food and incapability of achieving a sense of satiety, which makes adherence to a diet unfeasible, unless severe restriction of freedom is applied. Likewise weight control is a major challenge in these patients; progressive increase in weight usually occurs and the development of life-threatening complications of obesity is frequent. Troglitazone has proved to be effective in the treatment of hyperglycaemia and a few cases of bariatric surgery for the treatment of obesity have been reported. However, an effective treatment strategy has not yet been developed.

Commentary

This case clearly indicates that diagnosing type 2 diabetes in a young patient is not straightforward. Although this type of diabetes is rather common especially in the obese, a number of alternative hypotheses should be explored in the young, before the diagnosis is established. Likewise obesity starting in early childhood deserves medical attention and careful search for genetic defects. If not diagnosed in childhood, genetic syndromes of obesity may be easily misdiagnosed later in life, a careful history collection and clinical examination would help to avoid missing the correct diagnosis.

Further reading

1. Report of the Expert Committee on the Diagnosis and Classification of Diabetes Mellitus. *Diabetes Care* 1997; **20**: 1183–97.

2. Atterseley AT. Maturity-onset diabetes of the young: clinical heterogeneity explained by genetic heterogeneity. *Diabetic Med* 1998; **15**: 15–24.

3. Holm VA, Cassidy SB, Butler MG et al. Prader-Willi Syndrome: consensus diagnostic criteria. *Pediatrics* 1993; **91**: 398–402.

4. Young ID. Diagnosing Prader-Willi syndrome. *Lancet* 1995; **345**: 1590.

5. Schuster DP, Osei K, Zipf WB. Characterisation of alterations in glucose and insulin metabolism in Prader Willi subjects. *Metabolism* 1996; **45**: 1514–20.

6. Bassali R, Hoffman WH, Chen H, Tuck-Muller CM. Hyperlipidemia, insulin-dependent diabetes mellitus and rapidly progressive diabetic retinopathy and nephropathy in Prader-Willi Syndrome with deletion (15) (q11.2q13). *Am J Med Genet* 1997; **71**: 267–70.

CASE 17: HOW THE EYES HABITUATE TO THE CHANGING APPEARANCE OF THE PATIENT: THE ADVANTAGE OF A FRESH LOOK

Arno WFT Toorians, Robert J Heine and
Michaela Diamant

History

A 53-year-old woman was referred to the Department of Endocrinology at the
University Hospital for a second opinion because of failure to control her diabetes
and hypertension in spite of an extensive long-term effort. The referring physician
wrote with understatement that 'he seldom referred patients to a university
hospital for problems of this kind, however, in this case he would not like to
withhold the patient the benefit of the excellent care of skilled university
diabetologists'.

She had a medical history of a melanoma excision and varicose veins surgery.
Type 2 diabetes mellitus was discovered at the age of 40 years, preoperatively
before the latter operation. After initial treatment with sulphonylurea derivatives
(SUD), insulin therapy was added and finally she was treated with SUD and
intensive insulin therapy consisting of four injections: an intermediate-acting
insulin at night-time and three preprandial injections of an insulin analogue. For
the last 2 years, her glycated haemoglobin (HbA1c) levels had ranged between
11% and 15%, with random plasma glucose levels varying between 7 and
21 mmol/L. Continuous subcutaneous insulin infusion therapy was proposed
repeatedly at the referring clinic. However, the patient kept refusing this form of
therapy. Blood pressure values ranged from 180 to 200 mmHg (systolic) and 90
to 105 mmHg (diastolic), in spite of triple therapy consisting of an angiotensin-
converting enzyme inhibitor, a thiazide diuretic and a centrally acting
antihypertensive drug.

She complained of progressive fatigue, loss of physical fitness and sleeplessness
during the previous 2 years. She suffered from attacks of hot flushes and sweating
which she ascribed to a menopausal state, as she stopped menstruating at the age
of 48 years. Hypoglycaemia was excluded repeatedly. Her visual acuity was good
and the most recent ophthalmologic check-up, including fundoscopy, did not
reveal any abnormalities. She had experienced a weight gain of 3 kg during the
last few years, which she ascribed to smoking cessation. There was no history of

alcohol abuse. There was no apparent reason to question her compliance to treatment prescriptions. Her current insulin regimen consisted of a total dose of 110 U per 24 h.

Examination and investigations

At physical examination a plethoric face and centripetal adiposity were noted, but no buffalo hump. The patient was obviously sweating. Her weight was 93 kg, her height 174 cm. Sitting blood pressure averaged 195/105 mmHg, and the pulse rate was regular with 110 beats per minute. The skin of both forearms showed eczematous lesions and she mentioned that these itching spots healed slowly. The skin of the abdomen showed no abnormalities at the insulin injection sites, no striae or bruises. Further examination, including neurological testing, was unremarkable.

Diagnosis

The patient was referred to a diabetes educator and a dietician to evaluate her diet and energy intake. Initial laboratory examination revealed normal ESR, haematological and biochemical parameters. HbA1c was 11.1% (reference values: 4.3–6.1%). A random serum cortisol taken at midday was 630 nmol/L (ULN for early morning cortisol: 600 nmol/L). A 24-h urine collection contained an elevated level of free cortisol (606 nmol/L; normal range: 30–270 nmol/24 h), which was confirmed in additional collections (435 and 897 nmol cortisol and 4.8 and 5.0 nmol creatinine per 24 h, respectively). Subsequent determination of an early morning plasma ACTH level was 5.6 pmol/L (normal: 2–12 pmol/L), indicating autonomous ACTH production. A dexamethasone suppression test (7 mg administered intravenously over 7 h) showed suppression of cortisol from 705 to 89 nmol/L, further confirming the suspected central cause of the Cushing's syndrome. An MRI examination of the pituitary gland showed enlargement of the adenohypophysis with two nodular lesions (with diameters of 3 and 6 mm, respectively) located at the left side and the medial line, respectively, compatible with the diagnosis of a corticotrope microadenoma (Hardy classification grade I).

Treatment and outcome

The patient consented to the proposed neurosurgical removal of the tumour. Preoperative bone densitometry was normal. Before neurosurgery, glycaemic and blood pressure control were optimized. Thus, metformin (1500 mg daily) was started and the insulin regimen was changed to two injections of intermediate-acting insulin (total dose 120 U/per 24 h), resulting in an HbA1c of 10%. Hypertension was treated by adding the long-acting calcium receptor antagonist amlodipine to the regimen, and blood pressure dropped to 160/90 mmHg. Then, the patient developed ankle oedema and painful feet, which showed no abnormalities on repeated examination. Non-steroidal anti-inflammatory drugs did not relieve the pain. Since amlodipine was suspected as the cause of the ankle oedema, no further diagnostic procedures were undertaken before surgery.

An uncomplicated transsphenoidal operation was performed with removal of the pituitary tumour. Immunohistological examination confirmed the diagnosis of an ACTH-producing pituitary adenoma as the cause of the Cushing's syndrome. Postoperatively, hydrocortisone replacement therapy was tapered successfully. Despite adjustment of the insulin dose the patient developed hypoglycaemic episodes. The total dose was further reduced to 80 U per 24 h, consisting of two injections of an intermediate-acting insulin daily. Within 4 weeks the HbA1c dropped to 8.2%. Blood pressure was easily controlled with a single daily dose of 5 mg enalapril to an average 140/80 mmHg. Despite discontinuation of amlodipine, her feet remained swollen and the gait was impaired. Now, the feet appeared warm and careful inspection revealed that both feet were wider and externally rotated, while standing, with a flattening of the arch. X-ray examination revealed osteopenia and alterations of the joint spaces. The diagnosis of bilateral Charcot's joint disease was made, which was treated with immobilization by means of casts.

What did I learn from this case?

This case, in the first place, illustrates how a fresh (clinical) view on a patient by a new physician may lead to solution of a long-standing problem, which through its gradual development had 'blurred' the vision of the initial doctor. The referring physician repeatedly had tried to motivate the patient, who showed all signs of the metabolic syndrome, to improve her glycaemic control. While doing this he overlooked the gradual development of the physical stigmata of Cushing's disease.

As a second lesson, this case demonstrates that our preoccupation with persisting treatment hurdles may narrow our diagnostic view with regard to newly emerging difficulties. The doctor responsible for this second opinion focused primarily on the diagnosis of pituitary adenoma causing Cushing's disease and the organization of the neurosurgical treatment. In the postoperative phase, when the patient improved clinically, the neuropathic arthropathy became apparent. Although ankle oedema is compatible with the use of dihydropyridine calcium channel-blockers, warm and functionally impaired painful feet with flattened arches in a patient with long-standing diabetes should have triggered the diagnosis of Charcot's arthropathy, which warrants immediate therapy.

CASE 18: A LARGE DOSE OF BEDTIME INSULIN — WHY?

Hannele Yki-Järvinen and Katriina Nikkilä

Background

Given that the history of treating patients with type 1 diabetes with insulin is much longer than that of patients with type 2 diabetes, some of us may be unfamiliar with the remarkable inter-individual variation encountered when treating patients with type 2 diabetes with insulin, as illustrated by the following case.

History

This 54-year-old man had a family history of both hypertension (mother) and type 2 diabetes (father) and was diagnosed as having essential hypertension at the age of 44 years. At this time, his fasting glucose was normal (5.6 mmol/L) and he weighed 120 kg (BMI 30 kg/m^2). Because of a high concentration of haemoglobin (190 g/L), an abdominal ultrasound was performed. The spleen was normal. The liver was perhaps slightly enlarged and possibly fatty. The patient used 'moderate amounts' of alcohol and smoked a packet of cigarettes a day. At a follow-up examination a year later, fasting glucose was 6.6 mmol/L. Three years later at the age of 47, the patient was admitted because of deep thrombosis in the right leg and was found to have diabetes with a fasting glucose of 13.9 mmol/L. Body weight was now 129 kg (BMI 32.2 kg/m^2). Serum triglycerides were 2.3 mmol/L. Glibenclamide was started at 1.75 mg × 2. Three years later, at the age of 50 years, the patient still weighed 129 kg despite attempts to lose weight, and had an HbA1c of 9.1% using glibenclamide 3.5 mg × 2 and metformin 500 mg × 2. Later the same year and over the next 2 years, HbA1c averaged 9.9%. No change was made in the medication. Blood pressure was well controlled with enalapril 20 mg and hydrochlorothiazide 25 mg and averaged 130/85 mmHg.

At the age of 53 years after being in poor glycaemic control ever since the clinical diagnosis of diabetes had been made 6 years earlier, insulin therapy was started with bedtime NPH and metformin. HbA1c was now 12.4% (reference range 4.0–6.0%) and body weight had decreased – possibly because of insulin deficiency and glucosuria – to 118.7 kg (BMI 29.7 kg/m^2). Glibenclamide was discontinued and metformin was continued at a dose of 2 g per day. The patient was instructed to inject 10 units of NPH insulin at bedtime and was given

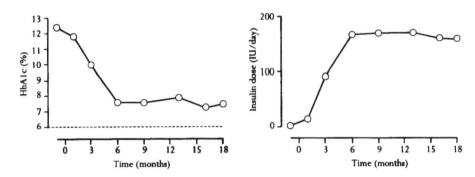

Figure 1 *Changes in HbA1c and insulin dose after start of treatment with bedtime NPH and metformin.*

instructions to increase the insulin dose by 2 units every 3 days, if fasting glucose was above 6 mmol/L on three consecutive mornings, and by 4 units, if fasting glucose was above 8 mmol/L on three consecutive mornings. The patient followed this algorithm and when he came to a follow-up visit 2 months later he was using 90 units of bedtime NPH insulin (Figure 1). HbA1c was now 10%. The patient insisted on getting a second shot of insulin, while the doctor thought this was not necessary as long as the fasting glucose target had not been reached. A mutual decision was made to try another 3 months with the current regimen. The patient was instructed to keep increasing the bedtime NPH insulin dose until the fasting glucose target (6 mmol/L) was reached. After 3 months, the bedtime insulin dose averaged 154 units and HbA1c 7.6%. After 6 months, the insulin dose averaged 176 units and at 18 months, the insulin dose was essentially unchanged at 160 units and HbA1c was 7.5%. Body weight increased by a total of 3 kg during the first 12 months and remained stable thereafter. At the start of insulin therapy, serum triglycerides were clearly elevated and averaged 3.4 mmol/L, HDL cholesterol was low (0.95 mmol/L) and LDL cholesterol was almost subnormal (1.3 mmol/L). At the end of 18 months of insulin therapy, serum triglycerides were normal (1.5 mmol/L), HDL cholesterol was still subnormal (0.85 mmol/L) and LDL cholesterol was normal (2.5 mmol/L).

Commentary and further examinations

This man already had several typical features of insulin resistance including hypertension, moderate obesity, a low HDL cholesterol concentration and hypertriglyceridaemia before developing diabetes. He also had a rarely mentioned feature, which is often associated with insulin resistance, a suspicion of a fatty liver. Secondary polycythaemia was probably mainly due to heavy smoking, which he did stop before commencing insulin therapy.

When judged according to the recently revised criteria for diabetes, diagnosis was delayed for 3 years, i.e. the fasting blood glucose concentration of 6.6 mmol/L would nowadays (when the blood glucose concentration diagnostic of diabetes has been lowered to 6.1 mmol/L) be sufficient to establish the diagnosis. Had an oral glucose tolerance test been performed, the diagnosis of diabetes would most likely have been made on the basis of the 2-h value (fasting blood glucose > 10 mmol/L) at this time. Subsequently, diabetes was diagnosed when fasting glucose had increased to 13.9 mmol/L. Thereafter the patient failed to lose weight or to exercise and his hyperglycaemia was inadequately treated for 6 years until insulin therapy was finally started.

Why was combination therapy with bedtime NPH and metformin chosen? This simple regimen was chosen because studies comparing various insulin regimens have shown that (i) glycaemic control has been better or similar, never worse with insulin combination therapy than with insulin alone administered as multiple insulin injections (NPH and regular insulin three times per day) or as a twice-daily split mixed insulin;[1] (ii) weight gain is a concern in an obese patient and has been shown to increase with the number of insulin injections and with injection of NPH in the morning rather than in the evening;[1] (iii) metformin counteracts weight gain during insulin therapy.[2,3]

Why did the patient require so much insulin? The patient required 176 units of bedtime NPH in addition to 2 g of metformin to achieve as good glycaemic control as was possible with insulin combination therapy using NPH (on average 7.2% in the FINFAT study with bedtime NPH insulin and metformin after 1 year of treatment).[3] The mean dose in the FINFAT study in patients whose body index was 29 kg/m^2, age 60 years and whose HbA1c was lowered from 10 to 7.2% was 42 units of NPH insulin at bedtime. To determine the cause or pathophysiological correlate of the high insulin requirement, the patient participated in a study specifically aimed at defining causes of variation in exogenous insulin requirements.[4] In this study, insulin absorption was determined by following the increment in free insulin concentrations after a subcutaneous insulin injection and insulin action was determined by the euglycaemic insulin clamp technique. In addition, various parameters reflecting body adiposity and composition including measurements of body weight and percentage fat, visceral and subcutaneous fat by MRI, the waist to hip ratio, thickness of subcutaneous adipose tissue at the site of the insulin injection (ultrasound) and quantification of percentage liver fat (proton spectroscopy) were performed.[4]

Insulin was absorbed normally in this patient (Figure 2). The patient was, however, extremely resistant to insulin, as evidenced by poor suppression of serum FFA by insulin administered i.v. and s.c. (Figure 2) and a low glucose infusion rate required to maintain euglycaemia during hyperinsulinaemia compared with other type 2 diabetic patients who were at a similar level of glycaemic control and who were also treated with bedtime NPH insulin and metformin.

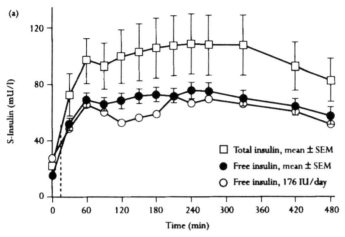

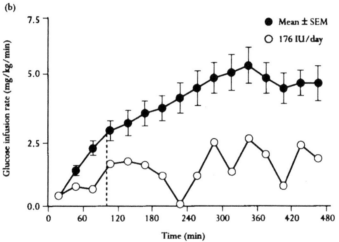

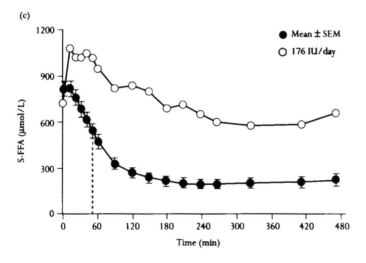

Figure 2
Absorption and action of s.c. insulin study. Serum free insulin concentrations (A), glucose infusion rate required to maintain euglycemia (B) and serum FFA (C) during the 480-min period after injection of a fixed dose of regular insulin s.c. The filled circles denote the mean values and the open circles the patient with an exceptionally high bedtime insulin dose (176 IU).

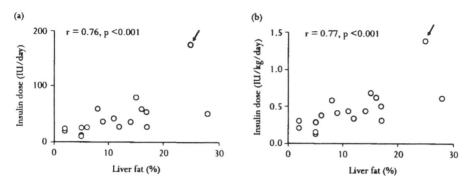

Figure 3 The relationship between percentage liver fat and insulin dose expressed as IU/day (A) and as IU/kg/day (B). The case discussed here is denoted with an arrow.

Glucose kinetic studies showed that the defect in insulin action was especially localized to the liver, which failed to suppress its glucose production normally during the exogenous insulin infusion. Furthermore, there was a very close correlation between the percentage of fat in the liver and suppression of glucose production by insulin, as well as between the percentage of fat in the liver and the daily insulin dose (Figure 3).

Is ectopic fat accumulation in the liver an underestimated cause of insulin resistance and a cause of high insulin requirements? Studies in ZIP1-fatless mice have demonstrated that ectopic fat accumulation in the liver and in skeletal muscle is associated with severe insulin resistance and signalling defects such as a defect in insulin-stimulated IRS-1 and IRS-2-associated PI 3-kinase activity.[5] Treatment of lipodystrophy in these mice by fat transplantation completely reverses insulin resistance.[6] This study thus demonstrated that fat deposition in an insulin-sensitive tissue causes insulin resistance in that tissue. The concept that subcutaneous adipose tissue is not necessary for the development of insulin resistance may also be applicable to humans, as various forms of lipodystrophy are accompanied by severe insulin resistance.[7] Also, accumulation of fat in skeletal muscle fibres has recently been shown to be associated with skeletal muscle insulin resistance and defect in activation of IRS-1-associated PI 3-kinase by insulin in normal men, independent of body mass index and body fat content.[8] Human data regarding the role of hepatic fat as an independent determinant of hepatic insulin resistance are sparse. This is probably in part because in the past it has been difficult to quantify hepatic fat without taking a liver biopsy. Proton spectroscopy provides a non-invasive tool that allows accurate quantification of hepatic fat with any standard MRI machine provided that the technical expertise required to analyse proton spectra is available.[4] When such expertise is not available, even slightly elevated alanine aminotransferase (ALT) concentrations may be indicative of a fatty liver. We have studied more than 100 non-diabetic individuals, who have had a 'non-alcoholic fatty liver', i.e. no evidence of causes of a fatty liver such as excessive alcohol consumption, or toxic, drug-induced, viral or autoimmune hepatitis. In these apparently healthy men and women, an upper limit of normal for ALT corresponds to 5% liver fat by proton spectroscopy (unpublished data). The 28% liver fat of the present patient described here is thus clearly abnormal and was the highest in the group of type 2 diabetic patients studied to determine the causes of variation in the insulin dose.

Even before the development of diabetes, the present patient, while undergoing an abdominal ultrasound examination because of a high haemoglobin concentration, was noticed to have a possible suspicion of a fatty liver and also had slightly elevated liver enzymes. It is of interest in this respect that abnormal liver function has recently been shown to be an independent predictor of diabetes. In 13,500 US adults aged 16–74 examined in the Third National Health and Nutrition Examination Survey (NHANES III), non-alcoholic fatty liver disease (NAFLD) was defined on the basis of the following criteria:[9] negative hepatitis B and C serologies, average daily alcohol intake < 2 drinks in women and < 3 in men, AST, ALT or GGT elevated above normal. Adults with NAFLD were significantly and more than twice as likely to develop diabetes as those without NAFLD, even after adjustment for body mass index, age, gender and race using logistic regression.[9] Similarly, in the Hispanic Health and Nutrition Examination Survey, elevated ALT activity was associated with a 3.0-fold increase in the risk of developing diabetes, after adjustment for body mass index, age and sex.[10]

The clinical implication of this case is first that good glycaemic control can be achieved even with a simple insulin regimen such as bedtime NPH and metformin, provided that the insulin dose is adequately titrated. Of note, had the patient not increased the dose by 2 units approximately every 3 days, it would not have been possible to increase the dose from 10 to 160 units in 6 months. If the dose adjustments had only been made in, for example, 5 unit increments at outpatient visits every 3 months, it would have taken 30 visits or 7.5 years to reach the glycaemic target. The second clinical implication might be that whenever we encounter elevated liver enzymes in a type 2 diabetic patient, we should not automatically attribute the increase to alcohol or obesity, although these are certainly common causes of abnormal liver function tests. We should consider the possibility that the elevated liver enzymes (which may include gamma-glutamyl transferase even in the absence of excessive alcohol consumption in addition to ALT or aspartate aminotransferase) may reflect NAFLD and accumulation of fat in the liver even in the absence of obesity. This, in turn, is likely to lead to higher than average hepatic insulin resistance and insulin requirements. Obviously, a fatty liver resulting from excessive alcohol consumption or obesity is also likely to be more insulin-resistant than a non-fatty liver.

References

1. Yki-Järvinen H. Combination therapies with insulin in type 2 diabetes. *Diabetes Care* 2001; **24**: 758–67.

2. Aviles-Santa L, Sinding J, Raskin P. Effects of metformin in patients with poorly controlled, insulin-treated type 2 diabetes mellitus. A randomized, double-blind, placebo-controlled trial. *Ann Intern Med* 1999; **131**: 182 8.

3. Yki-Järvinen H, Ryysy L, Nikkilä K, Tulokas T, Vanamo R, Heikkilä M. Comparison of bedtime insulin regimens in patients with type 2 diabetes mellitus. A randomized, controlled trial. *Ann Intern Med* 1999; **130**: 389–96.

4. Ryysy L, Häkkinen AM, Goto T et al. Hepatic fat content and insulin action free fatty acids and glucose metabolism rather than insulin absorption are association with insulin requirements during insulin therapy in type 2 diabetic patients. *Diabetes* 2000; **49**: 749–58.

5. Kim JK, Gavrilova O, Chen Y, Reitman ML, Shulman GI. Mechanism of insulin resistance in A-ZIP/F-1 fatless mice. *J Biol Chem* 2000; **275**: 8456–60.

6. Gavrilova O, Marcus-Samuels B, Graham D et al. Surgical implantation of adipose tissue reverses diabetes in lipoatrophic mice. *J Clin Invest* 2000; **105**: 271–8.

7. Reitman ML, Arioglu E, Gavrilova O, Taylor SI. Lipoatrophy revisited. *Trends Endocrinol Metab* 2000; **11**: 410–16.

8. Virkamäki A, Korsheninnikova E, Seppälä-Lindroos A et al. Intramyocellular lipid is associated with resistance to in vivo insulin actions on glucose uptake, antilipolysis and early signaling pathways in human skeletal muscle. *Diabetes* 2001; **50**: 2337–43.

9. Clark JM, Diehl A-MBFL. Nonalcoholic fatty liver disease and the risk of type 2 diabetes in the United States. *Diabetes* 2001; **50**: A38.

10. Meltzer AA, Everhart JE. Association between diabetes and elevated serum alanine aminotransferase activity among Mexican Americans. *Am J Epidemiol* 1997; **146**: 565–71.

CASE 19: TREATMENT OF INSULIN RESISTANCE IN TYPE 2 DIABETES

Martin Ridderstråle and Kerstin Berntorp

History

The patient, a 66-year-old overweight non-smoking woman suffering from type 2 diabetes since 1977, had been transferred from oral hypoglycaemic treatment to insulin in 1994 and had been admitted to hospital on several occasions because of dysregulated diabetes. Hyperlipidaemia, non-proliferative retinopathy, peripheral neuropathy and microalbuminuria were noted complications to her disease. She had suffered two myocardial infarctions and had been receiving pharmacological treatment for hypertension, hyperlipidaemia and congestive heart failure since 1997. In 1998 she underwent coronary bypass surgery and since then has stable angina pectoris. At previous repeated admissions for dysregulated type 2 diabetes fasting plasma glucose had been around 25 mmol/L despite repeated increases of insulin dose at home. In October 1999 she received an intravenous insulin infusion for 3 days to alleviate insulin resistance and was discharged with a daily insulin dose of 170 IU given four times daily. HbA1c at that time was 10.2% (corresponding to 11.0% in DCCT standard).

In February 2000 the patient was admitted to hospital for initiation of rosiglitazone treatment. Upon clinical investigation there were no signs of congestive heart failure. Her weight was 92 kg corresponding to BMI 35 kg/m², and resting blood pressure was 150/60 mmHg. Her total daily insulin dose was 176 IU given as short-acting insulin three times daily and medium-acting insulin at bedtime. Routine blood tests, including plasma creatinine and liver enzymes, were normal. HbA1c was 8.5% (9.4% DCCT standard) and plasma lipids were slightly elevated. After 1 week the patient was discharged with no further changes in treatment other than rosiglitazone added 4 mg twice daily to previous insulin therapy (total dose 174 IU). The ensuing treatment was managed together with the district nurse and the patient's general practitioner. After only 1 week pendulant blood glucose profiles (3–16 mmol/L) were reported and the patient had experienced several hypoglycaemic episodes. In a few days the prescribed daily dose of insulin was reduced to 138 IU and plasma glucose was stabilized at around 8 mmol/L.

One month after rosiglitazone had been introduced the patient complained of painful peripheral oedema and breathlessness (dyspnoea) and diuretic treatment was reinforced (furosemide from 250 to 500 mg daily). Two months later the patient returned to the outpatient clinic. She now had an increase in plasma creatinine to 142 μmol/L, a decrease in HbA1c to 5.4% (6.4% DCCT standard) and a marked decrease in albumin excretion rate from 1379 to 150 μg/min. Because of worsening congestive heart failure, diuretic treatment was further reinforced and the patient was transferred to the Cardiology Department. Her condition stabilized temporarily but a few weeks later, after 4 months of treatment, rosiglitazone had to be withdrawn. The HbA1c level at this point was 5.3% (6.3% DCCT standard). The insulin regimen was once again re-evaluated and she was prescribed a mixture of short- and long-acting insulin, which was titrated on an outpatient basis up 186 IU daily.

Two months after the discontinuation of rosiglitazone the patient was admitted again to the hospital because of poor glycaemic control and diabetic symptoms. Her HbA1c was again 10.3% (11.1% DCCT standard), plasma creatinine was 149 μmol/L and plasma lipids were moderately elevated. Albumin excretion had decreased further to 99 μg/min. Liver enzymes were normal. The patient was prescribed metformin 500 mg twice daily as a complement to her insulin treatment. One month later HbA1c was somewhat reduced to 8.7% (9.6% DCCT standard) but the metformin treatment had to be discontinued because of progressive renal failure with increasing creatinine and urea levels.

Commentary

Type 2 diabetes is characterized by both peripheral and hepatic insulin resistance.[1] In most patients glucose levels continue to rise despite treatment with insulin, sulphonylureas or metformin.[2] The thiazoledinediones (TZDs) represent a new principal class of drugs for treatment of type 2 diabetes. They selectively reduce peripheral insulin resistance and this effect is more pronounced than that seen with biguanides. TZDs bind to and activate the adipocyte-specific transcription factor peroxisomal proliferator-activated receptor gamma (PPARγ) which together with the retinoic acid receptor X bind to specific gene sequences and increase their transcription in adipocytes.[3-7] Unlike the first-generation TZD troglitazone, which had to be withdrawn from clinical practice because of severe side-effects in the liver, no such adverse events have been reported for the second-generation preparations (rosiglitazone and pioglitazone) that have now been introduced in the USA and Europe. However, congestive heart failure constitutes an absolute contraindication, as TZDs have been shown to cause fluid retention in clinical trials. The patient described above had been treated with various oral hypoglycaemic agents before being given multiple injections of high doses of insulin. Despite high daily doses of insulin her blood glucose profiles and HbA1c remained unacceptably high. Her insulin resistance could be overcome by intravenous insulin infusion but the effect was short-lasting. Despite the

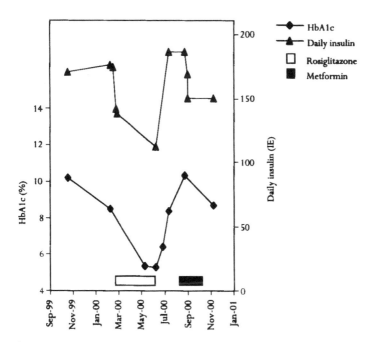

Figure 1 *HbA1c and prescribed daily insulin dose over time during treatment with rosiglitazone (4 mg × 2) and metformin (500 mg × 2).*

contraindications her metabolic deterioration was considered serious enough to warrant TZD treatment. She responded remarkably well to the combined treatment with rosiglitazone and insulin (Figure 1) but also suffered severely from major side-effects with worsening of congestive heart failure. The treatment had to be discontinued and insulin resistance recurred. No deterioration of liver function was observed. The complete explanation as to why TZDs cause fluid retention is not known. Preclinical data show that TZDs cause retention of both sodium and water as a class effect. Insulin can also cause fluid retention, which in combination with increased utilization of carbohydrates may be part of the explanation for the weight gain seen in patients treated with TZDs and insulin.

References

1. Beck-Nielsen H, Groop LC. Metabolic and genetic characterization of prediabetic states. Sequence of events leading to non-insulin-dependent diabetes mellitus. *J Clin Invest* 1994; **94**: 1714–21.

2. United Kingdom Prospective Diabetes Study (UKPDS) Group. Intensive blood-glucose control with sulfonylureas or insulin compared with conventional treatment and risk of complications in patients with type 2 diabetes. *Lancet* 1998; **352**: 837–53.

3. Ibrahimi A, Teboul L, Gaillard L et al. Evidence for a common mechanism of action for fatty acids and thiazolidinedione antidiabetic agents on gene expression in preadipose cells. *Mol Pharmacol* 1994; **46**: 1070–6.

4. Kahn CR, Chen L, Cohen SE. Unraveling the mechanism of action of thiazolidiniediones. *J Clin Invest* 2000; **106**: 1305–7.

5. Vamecq J, Latruffe N. Medical significance of peroxisome proliferator-activated receptors. *Lancet* 1999; **354**: 141–8.

6. Auwerx J. PPARγ, the ultimate thrifty gene. *Diabetologia* 1999; **42**: 1033–49.

7. Desvergne B, Wahli W. Peroxisome proliferator-activated receptors: nuclear control of metabolism. *Endocr Rev* 1999; **20**: 649–88.

CASE 20: A CASE OF PARTIAL LIPODYSTROPHY

Lisa R Tannock and Alan Chait

History

A 50-year-old Caucasian woman was referred with possible Cushing's syndrome. She was diagnosed with type 2 diabetes mellitus at age 43, and started using insulin a year later. Her past medical history was remarkable for a diagnosis of acute pancreatitis at age 47, which was attributed to hypertriglyceridaemia (triglycerides = 79 mmol/L (7000 mg/dL)). She also had a history of hypertension, and developed coronary artery disease at age 47, which was treated by angioplasty.

At her initial consultation with endocrinology, the patient complained of constant abdominal pain, with frequent nausea and vomiting. Her diabetes was poorly controlled with a HbA1c of 10.9%, despite using > 150 U/day of insulin. She reported a lifelong pattern of central obesity with disproportionately slender extremities. She denied any muscle weakness. She reported a dietary intake that was very low in fat, due to her self-observation that high dietary fat worsened her abdominal pain.

Examination and investigations

The patient was an obese Caucasian woman who weighed 92.3 kg (203 lbs), with a height of 1.62 m (5 feet 4 inches), resulting in a body mass index of 34.9 kg/m². Her obesity was striking in that it was very centrally located, with remarkable paucity of fat on her extremities. There was a shelf-like demarcation where her truncal obesity started at the level of the buttocks, with no subcutaneous fat palpable distally (Figure 1). Examination of her upper extremities showed an absence of subcutaneous fat on her forearms bilaterally, but with a gradual appearance of fat in her high upper arms, such that subcutaneous fat did overlie her upper triceps. There was an abundance of subcutaneous fat under her chin, and on her face, and a noticeable dorsal hump. There was no hirsutism, and her abdominal striae were pale. Her skin was not atrophic, and there was no acanthosis nigricans. Her blood pressure was 160/90 bilaterally, and pulse rate was 68. Visual fields were full by confrontation. Thyroid examination was normal, and there was no lymphadenopathy. Abdominal examination demonstrated a diffusely tender abdomen, with no guarding or peritoneal signs. Hepatomegaly

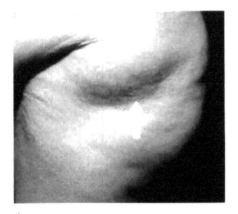

A

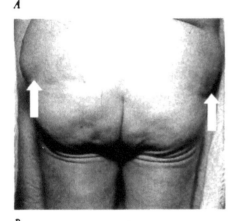

B

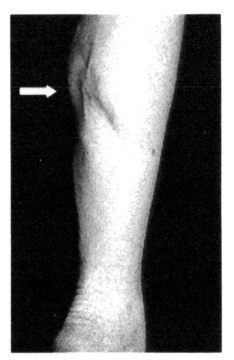

Figure 2 *Impression of calf muscle hypertrophy due to lack of subcutaneous adiposity.*

Figure 1 *Shelf-like demarcation where truncal obesity starts at the level of the buttocks (A, lateral view). Note absence of subcutaneous fat on upper thighs (B, posterior view).*

was demonstrated by a mid-clavicle span of 18 cm by percussion; however, the liver edge was not palpable due to her abdominal obesity. Neurological examination was normal, with normal reflexes, normal sensation to 5.09 g monofilament and normal proprioception. Muscle strength was normal including the ability to rise from a squatting position several times. She did have mild pitting oedema bilaterally distal to her knees. There was the impression of calf muscle hypertrophy, with clear outline of her muscular anatomy and a lack of subcutaneous adiposity (Figure 2). The rest of her examination was unremarkable.

A fasting lipid profile showed striking abnormalities: total cholesterol was 6.7 mmol/L (259 mg/dL), triglycerides were 38.8 mmol/L (3437 mg/dL) and HDL cholesterol was 0.6 mmol/L (22 mg/dL). LDL could not be calculated due to the severely elevated triglycerides. Her HbA1c was 10.9%, and her fasting glucose level was 14.8 mM (267 mg/dL).

Discussion

The initial differential diagnosis included Cushing's syndrome, polycystic ovary syndrome, or partial lipodystrophy syndrome. However, there were no physical stigmata of Cushing's syndrome, other than the central obesity. In particular, the lack of skin atrophy and her good proximal muscle strength were against this diagnosis. Moreover, her urine free cortisol was normal. There was no history of infertility or amenorrhoea, making polycystic ovary syndrome highly unlikely. Thus, based on her physical examination, a diagnosis of partial lipodystrophy was made.

Commentary

Lipodystrophies are syndromes of abnormalities in body fat distribution. Dunnigan et al originally described a family with complete absence of subcutaneous fat from the limbs and trunk with excessive face and neck adiposity.[1] Shortly afterwards, Kobberling et al described a family with complete absence of subcutaneous fat on limbs only, with normal fat on the face and trunk.[2] Other forms of lipodystrophy also have been described, including acquired lipodystrophy related to use of protease inhibitors for the treatment of HIV. The familial partial lipodystrophies as originally described by Kobberling and Dunnigan have been reclassified as limb lipodystrophy (type 1) or limb and trunk lipodystrophy (type 2).[3] The patient described in this report has features of type 1 or limb lipodystrophy, with absent subcutaneous fat on her limbs, and excessive truncal, face and neck adiposity. This syndrome often is associated with insulin resistance and difficult to control diabetes, marked hypertriglyceridaemia leading to complications such as pancreatitis, and premature cardiac disease, all of which were evident in this patient. However, not all patients with partial lipodystrophy have such extreme elevations in their triglycerides. Many of the cases of lipodystrophy reported are familial, but a few reports also suggest that sporadic cases exist. Recently mutations in the nuclear gene lamin A/C (LMNA) have been reported in Canadian kindreds with familial partial lipodystrophy type 2 (Dunnigan type).[4]

Treatment and outcome

Due to the extremely elevated triglycerides at the time of consultation the patient was immediately placed on a very low (< 5%) fat diet, and gemfibrozil 600 mg b.i.d. Her insulin dose was increased to improve glycaemic control. She required as much as 280 U/day of insulin, in divided doses, to reduce her HbA1c to 7.5%. This also helped the hypertriglyceridaemia. With this therapy, she remained free from pancreatitis; however, she gained 30 lb over the following 8 months. Because of the large dose of insulin required, and to counter the weight gain, rosiglitazone 4 mg and metformin 500 mg b.i.d. were added. The addition of these agents allowed a reduction in her total daily insulin dose from 280 U to 120 U/day. Over the subsequent year she had a 30 lb weight loss, and her HbA1c was maintained at 7.3%. Her lipid profile also improved significantly so that her total cholesterol was reduced to 4.1 mmol/L (160 mg/dL), triglycerides 5.2 mmol/L (464 mg/dL) and HDL cholesterol 0.85 mmol/L (33 mg/dL).

We recommend that all patients with difficult to control diabetes mellitus with central obesity, particularly if associated with hypertriglyceridaemia, be examined carefully for clinical evidence of partial lipodystrophy. In our experience these patients often are referred for consideration of Cushing's syndrome due to their physical experience. The clue to the diagnosis of partial lipodystrophy is the physical examination. Although the data on therapy and prognosis of this diagnosis are limited at present, our experience suggests that aggressive lipid-lowering therapy, combined with use of insulin-sensitizing agents, may improve the metabolic profile of these patients, which hopefully in time will result in improved outcomes.

References

1. Dunnigan MG, Cochrane MA, Kelly A, Scott JW. Familial lipoatrophic diabetes with dominant transmission: a new syndrome. *Q J Med* 1974; **49**: 33–48.

2. Kobberling J, Willms B, Katterman R, Creutzfeldt W. Lipodystrophy of the extremities. A dominantly inherited syndrome associated with lipoatrophic diabetes. *Humangenetik* 1975; **29**: 111–20.

3. Kobberling J, Dunnigan MG. Familial partial lipodystrophy: two types of an X linked dominant syndrome, lethal in the hemizygous state. *J Med Genet* 1986; **23**: 120–7.

4. Cao H, Hegele RA. Nuclear lamin A/C R482Q mutation in Canadian kindreds with Dunnigan-type familial partial lipodystrophy. *Hum Mol Genet* 2000; **9**: 109–12.

CASE 21: SEVERE INSULIN RESISTANCE

David Savage and Stephen O'Rahilly

History

The patient, a 56-year-old woman, initially presented with oligomenorrhoea and hirsutism at the age of 19 years. Subsequent difficulties with conception were successfully managed with ovulatory induction therapy, but her first pregnancy (age 25 years) was complicated by gestational diabetes and pre-eclampsia. Diabetes persisted after the pregnancy and although dietary modification and oral anti-hyperglycaemic therapy were tried, she required insulin by the age of 30. A second pregnancy (age 32 years) was again complicated by severe pre-eclampsia with fetal loss. Hypertension persisted after this pregnancy, necessitating the institution of antihypertensive therapy. Despite increasing insulin doses her diabetic control remained suboptimal and she developed microvascular complications. Her therapy included 280 U insulin daily and four antihypertensive agents.

Examination and investigations

On examination she was hirsute, with acanthosis nigricans in the axillae and at the base of the neck. Her body mass index was normal ($24.4\,kg/m^2$), but her waist:hip ratio was elevated at 1.1 (normal value (N) < 0.86). This was primarily due to a reduction in limb and gluteal fat with preservation of truncal fat (Figure 1). She had prominent peripheral veins and well-defined peripheral musculature, which considering that she did very little exercise was particularly noteworthy. Her blood pressure remained elevated at 180/80. She had no detectable features of liver disease. She had bilateral diabetic retinopathy, proteinuria and peripheral neuropathy, but no clinical evidence of peripheral macrovascular disease.

Biochemical tests revealed diabetic dyslipidaemia (triglycerides, 5.7 mmol/L; HDL, 0.58 mmol/L; LDL, N), hyperuricaemia (0.38 mmol/L (N = 0.15–0.35 mmol/L)) and altered liver function tests (ALT, 85U/L (N < 50 U/L); GGT, 68 U/L (N < 51 U/L); ALP, N). Abdominal ultrasound findings of a diffuse increase in hepatic echogenicity were consistent with fatty liver (non-alcoholic steatohepatitis).

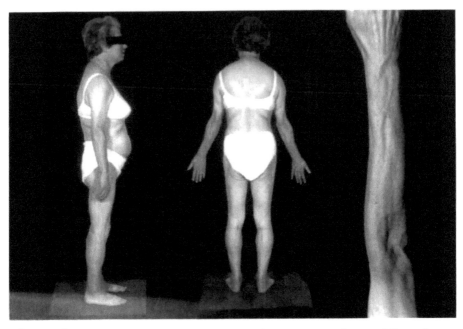

Figure 1 A 56-year-old woman with severe insulin resistance and a novel form of partial lipodystrophy secondary to a mutation in PPARγ.[5] Note the paucity of gluteal and limb fat with preservation of truncal fat.

Diagnosis

In summary this patient had early-onset type 2 diabetes with features of the HAIR-AN (hyperandrogenism, insulin resistance and acanthosis nigricans) syndrome. Hypertension, dyslipidaemia and hyperuricaemia completed the cluster of abnormalities known as syndrome X. Non-alcoholic steatohepatitis (NASH) was the most likely explanation of her hepatic dysfunction, as she consumed < 2 units of alcohol per week, was not taking any hepatotoxic drugs and, hepatitis B and C serology were negative.

Commentary

Type 2 diabetes mellitus (T2DM) is the result of two physiological defects: resistance to the metabolic actions of insulin combined with defective insulin secretion. Which of these constitutes the primary insult is controversial in most patients with T2DM. Occasionally, however, one or other defect clearly predominates. MODY2 (maturity onset diabetes of the young type 2), an autosomal dominant condition caused by mutations in glucokinase, is one example of a condition primarily inducing β-cell dysfunction. HAIR-AN syndrome on the other hand, is one of the conditions principally characterized by severe peripheral insulin resistance. Other conditions included in this somewhat loosely defined entity of 'severe insulin resistance syndromes' include type A and B syndromes of severe insulin resistance, pseudoacromegaly and Rabson-Mendenhall syndrome.[1,2] While T2DM is generally thought to be polygenic in origin, severe insulin resistance syndromes appear to be monogenic in many cases and genetic studies are beginning to yield intriguing insights into the molecular mechanisms responsible for these syndromes.[3,4] In fact, genetic studies of the subject of this report led to the identification of a dominant negative mutation in the nuclear hormone receptor, peroxisome proliferator-activated receptor gamma (PPARγ).[5] This mutation was also found in her son, who has diabetes, hypertension, hyperuricaemia and NASH. PPARγ is a key transcription factor in adipogenesis[6] and, as this case illustrates, it also appears to be involved in the development of the metabolic disarray seen in syndrome X. Furthermore, it is the target of the latest addition to the range of oral agents used in T2DM, namely the thiazolidinediones (TZDs).

Given PPARγ's central role in adipogenesis it is not surprising that magnetic resonance imaging of body fat distribution and DXA measurement of total body fat suggest that the subject of this report has a form of partial lipodystrophy. While the development of diabetes in people with reduced body fat (lipodystrophy) as well as in those with excess fat (obesity) is at first glance counterintuitive, both conditions can be viewed as a failure of adipocytes to serve as storage depots for excess energy in the form of triglycerides. The ensuing flux of fatty acids to liver, muscle and β-cells may be central to the subsequent development of peripheral insulin resistance, β-cell dysfunction and diabetes.[7]

Learning points

1. Recognition of T2DM as a heterogeneous syndrome and of the potential importance of the interplay between fatty acid and glucose metabolism in its pathogenesis.
2. For practical purposes severe insulin resistance should be considered in patients with acanthosis nigricans and a fasting insulin level > 200 pmol/L. Diabetic dyslipidaemia, hypertension, NASH, menstrual disturbances (in women) and cosmetic problems (acanthosis nigricans and hirsutism) are also commonly noted in these syndromes and should be screened for and treated where possible, in all cases.
3. Awareness of lipodystrophies and other syndromes of severe insulin resistance. While these syndromes are rare, their recognition may well prove to be of therapeutic benefit to individual patients. For example, patients with total lipodystrophy may improve dramatically with leptin therapy.[8]

References

1. Tritos NA, Mantzoros CS. Clinical Review 97: syndromes of severe insulin resistance. *J Clin Endocrinol Metab* 1998; **83**: 3025–30.

2. Garg A. Lipodystrophies. *Am J Med* 2000; **108**: 143–52.

3. Baynes KCR, Whitehead J, Krook A, O'Rahilly S. Molecular mechanisms of inherited insulin resistance. *Q J Med* 1997; **90**: 557–62.

4. Shackleton S, Lloyd DJ, Jackson SN et al. LMNA, encoding lamin A/C, is mutated in partial lipodystrophy. *Nat Genet* 2000; **24**: 153–6.

5. Barroso I, Gurnell M, Crowley VEF et al. Dominant negative mutations in PPARγ associated with severe insulin resistance, diabetes mellitus and hypertension. *Nature* 1999; **402**: 880–3.

6. Willson TM, Brown PJ, Sternbach DD, Henke BR. The PPARs: from orphan receptors to drug discovery. *J Med Chem* 2000; **43**: 527–50.

7. Bergman RN, Ader M. Free fatty acids and pathogenesis of type 2 diabetes mellitus. *Trends Endocrinol Metab* 2000; **11**: 351–6.

8. Oral EA, Simha V, Ruiz E et al. Leptin-replacement therapy for lipodystrophy. *N Engl J Med* 2002; **346**: 570–8.

CASE 22: TYPE 2 DIABETES MELLITUS — ORIGINS IN CHILDHOOD?

Russell S Scott

History

A 13-year-old Caucasian girl had dermatology review for treatment of granuloma annulare on one of her ankles. Triamcinolone was injected intradermally and blood tests were requested for haematology and basic biochemistry. The blood samples were finally collected 6 days after the steroid injection and showed a raised random glucose level of 14.9 mmol/L.

Apart from the granulomatous skin lesion, there was no significant past history. The patient was a middle child of a business couple. An aunt of the mother had diabetes mellitus, and although the mother did not have diabetes mellitus at this time, it was subsequently diagnosed 6 years later. The patient was a bright student, excelling academically at school. She enjoyed a range of extracurricular activities, including indoor and outdoor sports. She was using no medications upon presentation.

Examination and investigations

At medical review the subject was a well looking, markedly overweight, pre-pubertal girl, Tanner stage III. Height was 166 cm (90th percentile) and weight 77.8 g, BMI 28.2. Other clinical examination was unremarkable. Capillary blood glucose at this review in the afternoon was 3.9 mmol/L. Urinary ketones were negative. 75-g glucose tolerance testing was undertaken, confirming diabetes mellitus with fasting glucose 7.7 mmol/L and 2-h value 15.6 mmol/L.

Diagnosis

By far the most common diabetes disorder in this age group is type 1 autoimmune diabetes mellitus and this was considered the likely diagnosis, the assumption being that early detection had been made by serendipitous blood testing and that with passage of time metabolic decompensation would occur. It was presumed that the triamcinolone may have also been contributory to the hyperglycaemia. However, as the other biochemistry became available (Table 1) diagnostic reassessment and further investigation was necessary. Acromegaly and

Table 1   Initial biochemistry results

Parameter	Results	Normal range
Liver tests		
GGT (U/L)	283	< 50
ALT (U/L)	544	< 40
AST (U/L)	2.5	< 40
Islet cell antibodies	Negative	–
Fasting insulin (pmol/L)	654	< 75
HbA1c (%)	5.9	< 6.0

Cushing's syndrome were excluded. Islet cell antibodies were negative with human pancreatic (blood group 0) tissue; GAD and IA2 were not available as assays at this time and insulin antibodies were not detectable. Liver ultrasound was undertaken and this suggested fatty infiltration of the liver.

These data suggested that autoimmune-based type I diabetes was very unlikely and she was reclassified as having an insulin-resistant type 2 disorder.

Treatment and outcome

She was initiated to self-glucose measurement and a strategy of exercise and dietary adjustment was used to enhance insulin sensitivity. The patient remained committed to regular exercise and repeated reviews suggested that there was a good level of compliance to diet. Over the next 3 years she was monitored biochemically and clinically at 6-month intervals (Table 2). She went through menarche approximately a year after diagnosis at the age of 14½. By the age of 15, the insulin-resistant clinical features were much more marked. She had increased weight despite concerted efforts to limit progression. Insulin-resistant features were skin thickening, particularly over the bony prominences, and minor pigmentation (early acanthosis) in the skin creases around the neck and in the armpits. By this time she had developed a few striae in the abdomen as a consequence of the weight increase. Facial acne was present. Clinical and biochemical features of PCO were present. GGT and transaminase levels persisted approximately twofold above upper normality.

Metformin was initiated at age 16. GI intolerance limited the dose to 500 mg twice a day. On this therapy (Table 29.2) the liver function tests and insulin levels fell close to upper limits of the normal range. Over the subsequent next few years the intake of metformin was highly variable because of associated gastrointestinal difficulties. Self-monitored blood glucose levels were usually in the range 5.0–9.0 mmol/L, HbA1c levels 6.0–6.2%. Urinary albumin levels have never been elevated.

Table 2 Results of monitoring

Parameter	Age (years)							
	13.5	14	14.5	15	16.5	17.5	19.0	22.5
Time since presentation (years)	0	0.5	1	1.5	3	4	5.5	9
Treatment		Diet and exercise			Metformin started	Metformin	Nil	Metformin
Weight (kg)	78.5	81.2	91.0	89.7	92.2	100.3	113.1	104.6

Commentary

This case provides an opportunity to observe the natural history of type 2 diabetes over nearly a decade, with expression of profound insulin-resistance in pre-pubertal years. Typically, type 2 diabetes mellitus is diagnosed in adulthood, at which point there is usually strong suspicion that the disorder will have been present already for some years. Without the critical blood test at or around the time of the triamcinolone injections for the granuloma annulare, it is highly likely that this person would have remained asymptomatic and possibly the diabetes may have remained unrecognized today, approximately a decade later. The main messages that are illustrated by this case are:

Learning points

- Insulin resistance may be triggered in childhood, setting the scene for subsequent development of diabetes. Type 2 diabetes mellitus is the endpoint of a metabolic disturbance that may be present for many years and can even be detected in childhood.
- Despite strenuous efforts to secure insulin-sensitizing strategies of weight loss and increased exercise, progression of the metabolic derangement and weight gain occurred.
- The case illustrates the effectiveness of metformin in reducing insulin levels and thus presumably improving insulin resistance. The identification of fatty infiltration in the liver and associated abnormal liver tests is a frequent accompaniment of insulin-resistant disorders and also improves with metformin. Glitazones are another available option.
- Nowadays pharmacological treatment with metformin would be introduced at the earliest possible stage, even if the patient was metabolically compensated and euglycaemic. The Diabetes Prevention Trial suggests that such strategies delay the inevitable metabolic decompensation from an insulin-resistant 'pre-diabetes' state to diabetes mellitus.

Further reading

Despres JP, Lemieux I, Prud'homme D. Treatment of obesity: need to focus on high risk abdominally obese patients. *BMJ* 2001; 322: 716–20.

Gerich GE. The genetic basis of type 2 diabetes mellitus: impaired insulin secretion versus impaired insulin sensitivity. *Endocrinol Rev* 1998; 19: 491–503.

Kahn SE, Prigeon RL, Schwartz RS et al. Obesity, body fat distribution, insulin sensitivity and islet beta-cell function as explanations for metabolic diversity. *J Nutr* 2001; 131: 3545–605.

Lebovitz HE, Banerji MA. Insulin resistance and its treatment by thiazolidinediones. *Recent Progr Horm Res* 2001; **56**: 265–94.

Lewy VD, Danadian K, Witchel SF, Arglaniari S. Early metabolic abnormalities in adolescent girls with polycystic ovary syndrome. *J Pediatr* 2001; **138**: 38–84.

Mahler RJ, Adler ML. Type 2 diabetes mellitus: update on diagnosis, pathophysiology and treatment. *J Clin Endocrinol Metab* 1999; **84**: 1165–71.

CASE 23: TYPE 2 DIABETES IN CHILDHOOD

Robert S Lindsay and Peter H Bennett

History

Ms Y was seen at a routine health screening appointment with her mother. She is of full Pima Indian heritage, a Native American group who have lived in the southwestern United States for hundreds of years. In the Pima community, the National Institutes of Health offer screening for diabetes in all community members over the age of 5 years. Ms Y had no symptoms likely to be caused by diabetes. She did have a strongly positive family history. Her mother had developed type 2 diabetes at the age of 17 years (some 10 years before Ms Y was born) and went on to develop diabetic nephropathy requiring dialysis. Her father had developed diabetes in his mid-thirties. Three of Y's grandparents (at ages between 27 and 48) and three of her great-grandparents (at ages between 51 and 64) had also developed diabetes.

Examination and investigations

At the time of examination, Ms Y was 12½ years old. She was obese with height 152 cm, weight 76.0 kg (BMI 32.9 kg/m^2). Other physical examination was unremarkable apart from the presence of acanthosis nigricans. Plasma glucose was 5.6 mmol/L fasting and rose to 14.8 mmol/L 2 h after a 75-g oral glucose load. Other laboratory investigations included total cholesterol 4.4 mmol/L, triglycerides 1.3 mmol/L. Urinalysis showed heavy glycosuria and was dipstick negative for ketones, protein and blood. HbA1c was 5.8% (laboratory reference range 4.2–6.1%).

Diagnosis

The diagnosis is type 2 diabetes, a condition increasingly recognized in children and adolescents.[1] Type 1 diabetes should also be considered but is rare in Native American communities and made less likely by the absence of ketonuria. Tests for autoantibodies were negative in Ms Y, as is the case generally in Pima children with diabetes.[2] Maturity onset diabetes of the young (MODY) is another possible diagnosis. Originally described by Tattersall as diabetes with many clinical characteristics of maturity-onset (now termed type 2) diabetes but occurring in early life and with an of autosomal dominant inheritance in families, five different molecular causes of MODY have now been described. The pattern of diabetes incidence in Ms Y's family does not fit an autosomal dominant pattern and the causative mutations of MODY have not been found in the Pima community.[3]

Treatment and outcome

Ms Y was seen by paediatric services. She was counselled about the diagnosis of diabetes as well as treatment. She is currently managed by diet.

Commentary

Obesity and type 2 diabetes are increasing problems in childhood. While prevalence is higher in certain ethnic groups, including Native Americans, type 2 diabetes in childhood is by no means confined to these groups.[1] This case illustrates a number of important risk factors for the development of diabetes. Firstly, Ms Y was obese. The prevalence of obesity is rising in many countries, including in children, and undoubtedly contributes to the rising prevalence of type 2 diabetes. The definition of obesity in childhood is controversial. BMI, the most convenient, albeit indirect, clinical measure of body adiposity, is generally lower in children than adults.[4] Nevertheless, by any current criteria Ms Y was obese. Obesity in part acts by causing insulin resistance – an important determinant of diabetes risk[5] – which is also suggested by the presence of acanthosis nigricans. Thirdly, Ms Y's risk of diabetes was increased by intra-uterine effects of maternal diabetes. In the Pima community maternal diabetes increases the risk of both obesity[6] and type 2 diabetes[7] (Figure 1). Maternal diabetes is the most powerful predictor of type 2 diabetes in children and young people between the ages of 5 and 20.[8] Studies suggest that this influence is exerted by the intra-uterine environment.[7,9] The very early onset of type 2 diabetes in Ms Y will also place her children at increased risk of obesity and type 2 diabetes.[7]

Ms Y's family history of type 2 diabetes is of importance. Risk of diabetes in the Pima population is likely to have a large genetic component[10] and it is likely that Ms Y's family carries genetic variation predisposing to diabetes. In such families environmental factors will also be involved – it is notable that the age of onset of diabetes was in the sixth or seventh decade of life in Ms Y's great-grandparents and has fallen in succeeding generations. In part this may reflect influences of intra-uterine environmental effects as noted above, but it also indicates the more general environmental changes chiefly in diet, exercise and subsequent obesity that have led to increases in type 2 diabetes worldwide.

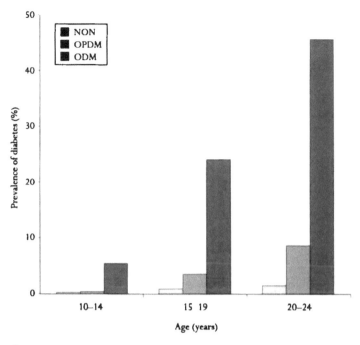

Figure 1 *Prevalence of diabetes in Pima Indian children. NON, offspring of non-diabetic mothers; OPDM, offspring of mothers who did not have diabetes at the time of pregnancy but subsequently developed type 2 diabetes; ODM, offspring of mothers with type 2 diabetes during pregnancy. (Redrawn from Pettitt et al.[7])*

Finally, Ms Y is a Pima Indian – an ethnic group with particularly high risk of obesity and type 2 diabetes. At first glance this might seem to make the case of Ms Y of less relevance to those not practising in Native American communities. Unfortunately, this is not the case. The Pima appear to be at the forefront of a trend to increasing obesity and type 2 diabetes in many populations and the recognition of these conditions in childhood.

What did I learn from this case?

This case reminds us of the potential for type 2 diabetes to occur even early in life and a number of important risk factors which increase this risk. One of these, her strong family history, gives clues to the probable important genetic component to the disease – and the hope that finding the cause of diabetes will lead to better prevention and treatment of, and perhaps even a cure for, type 2 diabetes. Family history should also be viewed from the patient's perspective. Patients like Ms Y have great reason to fear type 2 diabetes. They have observed the consequences of type 2 diabetes in their families and community and may view its onset almost as an inevitability. An abiding lesson is the burden that this places on patients like Ms Y and communities like the Pima.

How much did this case alter my approach to the care and treatment of my patients with diabetes?

Awareness of risk factors for type 2 diabetes may help us to diagnose disease early and avoid complications. In some communities, a high prevalence of disease may encourage community-wide screening. In other situations, particularly as obesity becomes a greater problem in childhood, awareness that the metabolic consequences of obesity may occur even early in life is critical.

Acknowledgements

We thank the members of the Gila River Indian Community for their continued support and participation in studies examining the causes, treatment and prevention of diabetes and obesity in their community.

References

1. Fagot-Campagna A, Narayan KM. Imperatore G. Type 2 diabetes in children. *BMJ* 2001; 322: 377–8.

2. Dabelea D, Palmer JP, Bennett PH, Pettitt DJ, Knowler WC. Absence of glutamic acid decarboxylase antibodies in Pima Indian children with diabetes mellitus. *Diabetologia* 1999; 42: 1265–6.

3. Baier LJ, Permana PA, Traurig M et al. Mutations in the genes for hepatocyte nuclear factor (HNF)-1alpha, -4alpha, -1beta, and -3beta; the dimerization cofactor of HNF-1; and insulin promoter factor 1 are not common causes of early-onset type 2 diabetes in Pima Indians. *Diabetes Care* 2000; 23: 302–4.

4. Cole TJ, Bellizzi MC, Flegal KM, Dietz WH. Establishing a standard definition for child overweight and obesity worldwide: international survey. *BMJ* 2000; 320: 1240–3.

5. Lillioja S, Mott DM, Spraul M et al. Insulin resistance and insulin secretory dysfunction as precursors of non-insulin-dependent diabetes mellitus. Prospective studies of Pima Indians. *N Engl J Med* 1993; 329: 1988–92.

6. Pettitt DJ, Knowler WC, Bennett PH, Aleck KA, Baird HR. Obesity in offspring of diabetic Pima Indian women despite normal birth weight. *Diabetes Care* 1987; 10: 76–80.

7. Pettitt DJ, Aleck KA, Baird HR, Carraher MJ, Bennett PH, Knowler WC. Congenital susceptibility to NIDDM. Role of intrauterine environment. *Diabetes* 1988; 37: 622–8.

8. Dabelea D, Hanson RL, Bennett PH, Roumain J, Knowler WC, Pettitt DJ. Increasing prevalence of Type II diabetes in American Indian children. *Diabetologia* 1998; 41: 904–10.

9. Dabelea D, Hanson RL, Bennett PH et al. Intrauterine exposure to diabetes conveys risk for diabetes and obesity in offspring above that attributable to genetics. *Diabetes* 1999; 48: A52.

10. Hanson RL, Elston RC, Pettitt DJ, Bennett PH, Knowler WC. Segregation analysis of non-insulin-dependent diabetes mellitus in Pima Indians: evidence for a major-gene effect. *Am J Hum Genet* 1995; 57: 160–70.

CASE 24: A 44-YEAR-OLD WOMAN WITH A HISTORY OF 20 YEARS OF 'BRITTLE TYPE 1 DIABETES'

John E Gerich

History

A 44-year-old woman was referred by her primary care physician for optimization of her diabetic control. She was first diagnosed with diabetes at age 24 because of symptoms of polyuria and polydipsia. These were recognized by the patient as possibly indicating diabetes since her mother and grandmother had developed the disease at about the same age. The patient had been treated with insulin from the start under the assumption that she had type 1 diabetes. The patient was currently on a regimen consisting of 7 units of 70/30 insulin before breakfast and lunch and 10 units of 70/30 insulin at bedtime. Although her HbA1c was 6.9%, she was bothered by frequent episodes of mild hypoglycaemia, which she attributed to small or delayed meals and to increased physical activity. She monitored her blood glucose levels erratically and did not carbohydrate-count or use an algorithm to adjust her insulin doses.

Past medical history was non-contributory except that she had had laser treatment for retinopathy in her right eye and a recent retinal detachment. She denied symptoms of thyroid and adrenal disease; her periods were regular. All of her three daughters also had diabetes starting in their teens which was being treated with insulin.

Examination and investigations

Physical examination was negative except for signs of laser therapy and decreased sensation and ankle jerks in both lower extremities suggestive of diabetic neuropathy. The patient was 5 feet 6 inches tall, weighed 140 lbs and had a blood pressure of 125/75 mmHg.

To maintain her good control, while reducing her hypoglycemia, the patient was placed on a basal bolus regimen consisting of 5 units of regular insulin prior to meals and 10 units of NPH at bedtime. She was given an algorithm for adjusting pre-meal doses based on pre-meal self-glucose monitoring and referred for diabetes education and nutritional counselling to learn carbohydrate counting. The laboratory tests shown in Table 1 were ordered and the patient was asked to return in 1 month for follow-up.

Table 1   Results of laboratory tests

Parameter	Patient's results	Normal values
Glucose	90 mg/dl	(65–110)
Sodium	142 meq/L	(135–145)
Chloride	107 meq/L	(98–108)
CO_2	27 meq/L	(22–31)
Potassium	4.5 meq/L	(3.4–4.7)
Creatinine	1.1 mg/dl	(0.7–1.1)
Calcium	9.2 mg/dl	(8.8–10.2)
Cortisol	16 mg/dl	(5–18)
TSH	2.6 MCU/ml	(0.30–5.00)
C-peptide	2.7 ng/ml	(0.9–4.0)
Creatinine clearance	92 ml/min	(87–107)
24-hr microalbuminuria	63 mg/24 h	(< 22)

Diagnosis

The plasma TSH and cortisol were ordered to exclude thyroid/adrenal insufficiency which may occur on an autoimmune basis in people with type 1 diabetes. The creatinine clearance and 24-h microalbuminuria were ordered to assess nephropathy, as the patient had evidence of retinopathy and neuropathy. The plasma C-peptide was ordered to confirm the diagnosis of type 1 diabetes, as the apparent dominant inheritance pattern of the diabetes and the low HbA1c on an insulin regimen inadequate for type 1 diabetes suggested that the patient might have maturity-onset diabetes of youth (MODY).

At follow-up visit, the patient reported preprandial glucose levels between 40 and 140 mg/dl with no improvement in frequency of hypoglycaemia. The results of the laboratory tests indicated no evidence of thyroid/adrenal insufficiency, but did indicate the presence of diabetic nephropathy. The plasma C-peptide of 2.7 ng/ml (normal 0.9–4.0) was considered to be incompatible with the diagnosis of type 1 diabetes and indicated that the patient probably had MODY.

Treatment and outcome

The patient was counselled about her type of diabetes and her nephropathy. She was started on an ACE inhibitor and was instructed to discontinue her pre-meal insulin and to take a combination of metformin and glyburide (2.5 mg/500 mg) twice daily along with her bedtime NPH. She was told to call back in 3–4 days with results of her self-glucose monitoring. As the patient did not call, she was called after 1 week. She stated that her pre-meal glucose values currently ranged between 87 and 129 mg/dl. She had discontinued her bedtime insulin on her own because of nocturnal hypoglycaemia.

At 3 months follow-up, her HbA1c was 6.7% (normal < 6.0%) and she had had no episodes of hypoglycaemia. She was grateful for getting off insulin and had called her daughters to have their type of diabetes checked.

Commentary

This case illustrates several points. Firstly, some patients with long-standing type 1 diabetes diagnosed before recognition of MODY may actually have MODY. Secondly, such patients may be successfully managed by oral agents despite many years of insulin treatment. Thirdly, MODY may be accompanied by the same microvascular complications as classic type 1 diabetes.

CASE 25: DIABETES IN HAIR-AN SYNDROME (HYPERANDROGENISM, INSULIN RESISTANCE AND ACANTHOSIS NIGRANS)

Elena Toschi, Alessandro Antonelli
and Ele Ferrannini

History

A 42-year-old woman was admitted because of poorly controlled diabetes. She had a positive family history of diabetes mellitus (father) and cardiovascular disease (mother). The patient was born prematurely (8 months) but had a normal psychosocial development until the age of 28 years, when she developed a bipolar (manic-depressive) syndrome. At 14, she had been admitted to another hospital to undergo tonsillectomy. Pre-operative evaluation revealed glycosuria (8–10 g/day) with normal fasting glucose levels. She had been prescribed a low-carbohydrate diet and glibenclamide (5 mg/day) and referred to our hospital. On that occasion, physical examination revealed a healthy looking girl, 154 cm tall and weighing 55 kg, with a feminine habitus and fine features. Menarche had not yet occurred. Her face and upper and lower extremities were moderately hirsute. The breasts were developed, and external genitalia were normal. The axillae and internal aspects of both thighs showed patches of accentuated skin folding with hyperpigmentation, consistent with areas of acanthosis nigricans, later confirmed by skin biopsy. Results of routine laboratory tests were within the normal limits and anti-nuclear antibodies were not detectable. Thyroid function test results were within normal limits. The glomerular filtration rate was 145 ml/min. Fundus oculi and electrocardiography were normal, as was the radiological appearance of the skull and sella turcica. Fasting plasma glucose was consistently below 4.0 mmol/L, but random postprandial readings ranged between 11 and 14 mmol/L. Glycosuria varied from 5–15 g/day, but ketone bodies were not found in the urine. On repeat determinations, fasting plasma insulin concentration exceeded 200 µU/mL (1200 pM), indicating severe insulin resistance. Anti-insulin and anti-insulin receptor antibodies were not found and binding of ^{125}I-insulin to circulating monocytes was normal.[1] The clearance of plasma insulin, as measured by a tracer technique,[2] was strikingly reduced (135 mL/min/m^2, normal 456 ± 22) in the presence of normal liver function. Despite the reduced clearance, fasting systemic insulin delivery rate was increased 10-fold (29.5 mU/min/m², normal 2.6 ± 0.3). The severe fasting hyperinsulinaemia – due to both reduced insulin clearance and insulin hypersecretion – associated with glucose intolerance, primary amenorrhoea, polycystic ovaries and hirsutism was characteristic of HAIR-AN syndrome with type C insulin resistance.[3] Three and half years later, the girl was admitted to a gynaecology department because of primary amenorrhoea and hirsutism. Marked male-pattern hirsutism and clitoromegaly were noted, the other external genitalia and secondary sexual characteristics were normal. At laparotomy, a highly hypoplastic uterus and white, enlarged polycystic ovaries were found. Ovarian wedge resection was performed. Two months later, menses appeared and returned, although irregularly, thereafter. Following surgery, insulin clearance increased to 264 mL/min/m² while insulin release decreased to 9.8 mU/min/m². The patient developed overt diabetes at age 35; compliance with anti-diabetic treatment and glycaemic control have been poor ever since.

Examination and investigations

On admission, physical examination revealed an overweight (body mass index = 27 kg/m²) patient with no signs of acanthosis nigricans or hirsutism. Fasting plasma glucose value was 16.7 mmol/L and HbA1c was 14% (normal up to 5.6%). Although plasma creatinine and blood urea nitrogen were normal, there was borderline microalbuminuria (211 mg/day) and marked dyslipidaemia (LDL-cholesterol 7.3 mM, triglycerides 3.5 mM, HDL-cholesterol 1.5 mM). Anti-IA2 and anti-GAD autoantibodies were not detectable. The fundus oculi presented plurifocal and flame-shaped haemorrhages and hard and cotton-wool exudates. The basal and exercise electrocardiogram and echocardiogram were normal, but on ultrasound there was an increase in intima-media wall thickness of the carotid bulb bilaterally.

Treatment and outcome

The patient was prescribed a hypocaloric diet, metformin, evening NPH insulin, a statin and 100 mg aspirin, and sodium valproate for her mental disturbance.

Commentary

HAIR-AN syndrome with type C insulin resistance is a rare form of primary, severe insulin resistance which is not accounted for by either the presence of anti-insulin receptor autoantibodies or a reduction in number of insulin receptors.

112

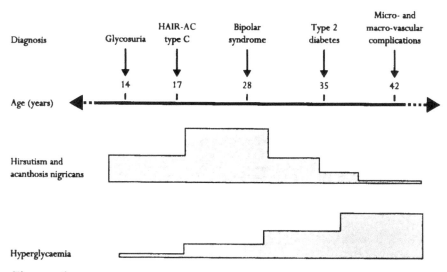

Figure 1 *Diagrammatic representation of aspects of the clinical course of the patient.*

The association with hyperandrogenism and polycystic ovaries is thought to result, at least in part, from the chronic hyperinsulinaemia. In fact, several lines of evidence[4] indicate that insulin stimulates ovarian thecal and stromal androgen secretion. In line with this in vitro evidence, mutations in the insulin receptor gene that cause severe hyperinsulinaemia are associated with ovarian hyperandrogenism, and, in some experimental models, manipulation of circulating insulin concentrations results in changes in circulating androgens.[5] In our patient, however, ovarian wedge resection resulted in an improvement of both the hyperandrogenism and the insulin resistance, suggesting that insulin and androgens may mutually interfere with one another. The origin of the acanthosis in HAIR-AN syndrome is uncertain. Acanthosis nigricans occurs in many conditions and, in a recent survey in Mexican Americans, appears to be under tight genetic control, as is its association with diabetes.[6] In this respect, the clinical course of our patient was remarkable in that glucose tolerance did deteriorate after years of insulin resistance and hyperinsulinaemia, but the acanthosis had spontaneously cleared by the time diabetes was clinically manifest (Figure 1). Moreover, our patient had a positive family history of diabetes, possibly accounting for the early manifestation and rather severe course of the disease (now evolving towards insulin deficiency with dyslipidaemia and micro- and macro-vascular complications). The mental disorder is also clinically relevant in our patient (previously described in association with the HAIR-AN syndrome),[7] because it limits her compliance with diabetes treatment and worsens her quality of life.

Learning points

In summary, the lesson from our case history is that the severe insulin resistance of HAIR-AN syndrome is a predecessor of early diabetes, especially, perhaps, against a background of genetic predisposition to diabetes, dyslipidaemia and premature atherosclerotic disease. This stands in contrast to the milder degrees of glucose intolerance usually found in women with polycystic ovaries, in whom morbidity and mortality from coronary heart disease are similar to those of the general population.[8] The acanthosis, on the other hand, may be transient and, other than attesting to the hyperandrogenism (and the interdependence of insulin action, insulin degradation and androgen secretion), its clinical impact remains uncertain.

References

1. Ferrannini E, Muggeo M, Navalesi R, Pilo A. Impaired insulin degradation in a patient with insulin resistance and acanthosis nigricans. *Am J Med* 1982; **73**: 148–54.

2. Ferrannini E, Cobelli C. The kinetics of insulin in man. I. General aspects. *Diabetes Metab Rev* 1987; **3**: 335–64.

3. Bar RS, Muggeo M, Roth J, Kahn CR, Havrankova J, Imperato-McGinley J. Insulin resistance, acanthosis nigricans, and normal insulin receptors in a young woman: evidence for a post-receptor defect. *J Clin Endocrinol Metab* 1978; **47**: 620–5.

4. Barbieri RL. Hyperandrogenism, insulin resistance and acanthosis nigricans. 10 years of progress. *J Reprod Med* 1994; **39**: 327–36.

5. Aquino Carlos P, Hernandez Valencia M. Insulin resistance in polycystic ovary syndrome. *Ginecol Obstet Mex* 1998; **66**: 446–51.

6. Burke JP, Duggirala R, Hale DE, Blangero J, Stern MP. Genetic basis of acanthosis nigricans in Mexican Americans and its association with phenotypes related to type 2 diabetes. *Hum Genet* 2000; **106**: 467–72.

7. Boor R, Herwig J, Schrezenmeir J, Pontz BF, Schonberger W. Familial insulin resistant diabetes association with acanthosis nigricans, polycystic ovaries, hypogonadism, pigmentary retinopathy, labyrinthine deafness, and mental retardation. *Am J Med Genet* 1993; **45**: 649–53.

8. Wild S, Pierpoint T, McKeigue P, Jacobs H. Cardiovascular disease in women with polycystic ovary syndrome at long term follow-up: a retrospective cohort study. *Clin Endocrinol* 2000; **52**: 595–600.

CASE 26: CALCIPHYLAXIS

Marie Degerblad and Maria Karlsson

History

A 65-year-old woman was referred to the Department of Dermatology at the Karolinska Hospital because of painful purple plaques on the abdominal wall, buttocks and thighs.

The patient had a morbid obesity (BMI 55 kg/m^2) and previous medical history of a thyroxine-substituted hypothyroidism. A year before the referral she was investigated because of increasing serum creatinine and albuminuria. The preliminary diagnosis was glomerulonephritis and a further diagnostic procedure with needle biopsy was planned. However, this was dismissed because of a 'silent' left kidney. Except for diuretics, treatment with active vitamin-D$_3$ was instituted because of high serum PTH values (500 ng/L). Further planned work-up was not fulfilled because the patient was then hospitalized several times owing to severe cardiac failure with atrial fibrillation and bouts of pulmonary oedema. Echocardiography revealed aortic and mitral valve stenosis and warfarin treatment was started.

Six months before referral to the Karolinska Hospital, painful violaceous indurations of the skin were noted for the first time. The primary locations of the indurations were the left breast and lower part of the abdominal wall. Erythrocyte sedimentation rate, C-reactive protein and plasma electrophoresis showed a marked inflammatory reaction. Concomitantly, the serum PTH level had increased to about 1000 ng/L.

During the following months, further skin areas were affected – thighs, buttocks and larger parts of the abdomen. During this period, the patient was investigated at a county hospital under the descriptive diagnosis 'paniculitis' with suggested aetiologies of lymphoma, scleroderma, collagenosis, pancreatic neoplasm or infection. Several biopsies of skin and muscles were performed with no conclusive diagnosis. In spite of thorough investigative procedures, a diagnosis could not be settled. Symptomatic treatment with glucocorticoids was started (prednisolone 20 mg/day) without any effect on the skin lesions. However, treatment was continued because the laboratory inflammatory markers decreased. During treatment, the patient became hyperglycaemic and insulin therapy was started while the prednisolone was reduced to 10 mg per day. Thereafter, an attempt with pulse treatment with cyclophosphamide was tried; this had no effect and treatment was finally withdrawn.

The subcutaneous lesions slowly progressed over time and became larger and more painful. Upon referral to the Department of Dermatology parts of the lesions were ulcerated with central necrosis. Parallel to this, general fluid retention and peripheral oedema progressed.

The continuing work-up revealed progressive renal failure with hypercalcaemia and hyperphosphataemia. Based on this, plus the clinical findings, the consultant endocrinologist and nephrologist suggested a diagnosis of calciphylaxis. In a retrospective evaluation of the biopsies taken earlier, a characteristic picture of medial calcification of small arteries in the subcutaneous tissue – calciphylaxis – could be demonstrated in a small fragment of one of the biopsies.

A decision to start haemodialysis was taken; however, during the preparation for this treatment, the patient died from acute pulmonary oedema.

Commentary

Calciphylaxis is a rare disorder appearing in patients with chronic renal failure. The onset of disease commences silently with a slowly developing calcification of subcutaneous arterioles (resistance vessels). Microscopically, calcium salts accumulate in the media of small arteries and arterioles, and the intima is thickened by loose connective tissue – primary lesions. These changes lead to diminishing lumen and later the development of secondary lesions with infarction of adjacent subcutaneous tissue and skin.[1]

The primary lesions in calciphylaxis are clinically silent. The secondary lesions give acute symptoms with painful violaceous and haemorrhagic mottling of the skin with tender induration of subcutaneous tissue mainly of the lower abdominal wall, breasts and thighs (central type) or more in the periphery on the arms and legs (peripheral type). Following this, patches of the skin ulcerate and expose necrotic adipose tissue. The necrosis usually progresses and serves as a portal of entry for potentially life-threatening infectious agents. There is no reliable treatment for stopping the progressive necrosis and the syndrome with central-type lesions is often lethal.[2] Treatment should always include attempts to correct serum calcium/phosphate imbalance and increased PTH levels; however, this is not easily achieved in these patients.[3] Skin debridement, haemodialysis and acute parathyroidectomy have been suggested as treatments.[4,5] None of these treatment modalities has been shown to be superior to the others.

With the above treatment, the peripheral type of the syndrome has a better prognosis. Our reported patient had several of the risk factors that have been suggested to relate to this syndrome: female gender, secondary hyperparathyroidism, obesity, oral anticoagulation and diabetes mellitus.[6]

According to the number of articles published in recent years, the number of patients with this rare disorder seems to be increasing, and several authors have reported patients with milder renal failure who developed the complete syndrome.[7] It is not clear whether this mirrors a true increase in incidence. An increased knowledge of this syndrome is important so that skin lesions characteristic for calciphylaxis can be identified earlier and hopefully treatment will be more successful.[1] As the syndrome is found more often in patients with diabetes and obesity, knowledge about the development of this clinical entity is mandatory for diabetologists.

Learning points

Characteristic laboratory findings are:
- Increased [Ca × phosphate] product
- Increased PTH level
- Increased sedimentation rate/C-reactive protein.

The suggested risk factors are:
- Obesity
- Diabetes mellitus
- Oral anticoagulation
- Female gender
- Secondary hyperparathyroidism.

Suggested treatments comprise:
- Correction of calcium/phosphate imbalance
- Ulcer treatment and revision
- Dialysis
- Acute parathyroidectomy.

References

1. Essary LR, Wick MR. Cutaneous calciphylaxis. An underrecognized clinicopathologic entity. *Am J Clin Pathol* 2000; 113: 280–7.

2. Janigan DT, Hirsch DJ, Klassen GA, MacDonald AS. Calcified subcutaneous arterioles with infarcts of the subcutis and skin ('calciphylaxis') in chronic renal failure. *Am J Kidney Dis* 2000; 35: 588–97.

3. Block GA. Prevalence and clinical consequences of elevated Ca × P product in hemodialysis patients. *Clin Nephrol* 2000; 54: 318–24.

4. Kriskovich MD, Holman JM, Haller JR. Calciphylaxis: is there a role for parathyroidectomy? *Laryngoscope* 2000; 110: 603–7.

5. Kang AC, McCarthy JT, Rowland C, Farley DR, van Heerden JA. Is calciphylaxis best treated surgically or medically? *Surgery* 2000; 128: 967–72.

6. Streit M, Paredes BE, Ruegger S, Brand CU. Typical features of calciphylaxis in a patient with end-stage renal failure, diabetes mellitus and oral anticoagulation. *Dermatology* 2000; 200: 356–9.

7. Smiley CM, Hanlou SU, Michel DM. Calciphylaxis in moderate renal insufficiency: changing concepts. *Am J Nephrol* 2000; 20: 324–8.

CASE 27: DIABETES AND HYPERCHYLOMICRONAEMIA IN AN HIV-POSITIVE MAN TREATED WITH ANTIRETROVIRAL THERAPY

D John Betteridge and Lisa Hamzah

History

A 45-year-old HIV-positive man presented to a sexual health clinic complaining of a 10-day history of thirst, polyuria and weight loss from 112 to 94 kg. He had been diagnosed HIV-positive after presenting with the ADS-defining diagnosis of cutaneous Kaposi's sarcoma 5 years previously. His father had type 2 diabetes. His antiretroviral therapy included ritonavir and saquinavir. Investigations showed a CD4 count of 340 and an undetectable viral load. His random blood glucose was 29.8 mmol/L, with plasma triglycerides of 116 mmol/L and cholesterol of 43.3 mmol/L. He was not acidotic.

Type 2 diabetes mellitus and hyperchylomicronaemia (type V hyperlipidaemia) were diagnosed against the background of a family history and protease inhibitor use. In view of the massive hypertriglyceridaemia, he was started on insulin together with high-dose omega-3 marine oils and fenofibrate. Some months later his HbA1c was 5.3% (<6%), triglycerides were 6.1 mmol/L and cholesterol was 5.9 mmol/L.

Despite his best endeavours to diet hard, his weight increased, and metformin 850 mg twice daily was introduced. His CD4 count began to drop, and his viral load increased to >45,000; a viral breakthrough, thought to be resistance to protease inhibitors, later confirmed by genetic testing, was diagnosed. His regime was changed to AZT, didanosine, nevirapine and abacavir. Some months later he presented to Casualty complaining of central crushing chest pain radiating to his left arm on exertion; a diagnosis of non-Q-wave myocardial infarction was made.

Two years post-diagnosis he was taking twice daily biphasic insulin and metformin with an HbA1c of 4.8%, plasma cholesterol 7.8 mmol/L and triglyceride 8.4 mmol/L. He was keen to reduce his insulin injections and was transferred to bedtime isophane insulin with continuation of metformin and addition of pioglitazone 30 mg. His latest biochemical profile includes HbA1c of 5.9%, cholesterol 6.2 mmol/L and triglyceride 4.7 mmol/L. His weight is 92 kg (BMI 28).

Discussion and learning points

Highly active antiretroviral therapy (HAART), usually combining nucleoside reverse transcriptase inhibitors with one or two protease inhibitors and/or a non-nucleoside reverse transcriptase inhibitor, is now considered standard treatment for HIV in the Western world.

Among the many well-documented side-effects of HAART, of most interest to the endocrinology are the common metabolic derangements.[1] These include lipodystrophy, affecting the face and peripheries and central fat accumulation, particularly intra-abdominally and over the dorsi-cervical spine. A number of metabolic abnormalities are common, including hypertriglyceridaemia, hypercholesterolaemia, insulin resistance, impaired glucose tolerance, overt type 2 diabetes mellitus and lactis acidaemia. Protease-inhibitor therapy has been implicated as the main cause of metabolic dysfunction, although body habitus changes and metabolic alterations have also been described with use of nucleoside reverse transcriptase inhibitors.[2,3]

There are important implications for patients diagnosed with these metabolic derangements. Of major concern is the possibility that the lipid disorders (often mixed lipaemia with low HDL cholesterol) contribute to premature coronary artery disease. This is highlighted in this case and there is emerging evidence in the literature.[4,5] However, large cohort studies will be necessary to quantitate coronary risk. In this case risk of pancreatitis from massive hypertriglyceridaemia is real. In addition, the psychosocial aspects of further diagnosis of chronic illnesses and poor body image from change in body habitus may lead to additional psychological difficulties.

The mechanisms for HAART-associated metabolic dysfunction appear to depend on a number of factors, including disease progression, combinations of antiretrovirals used, background metabolic profiles and genetics.[6] It is interesting to note that this patient also has a positive family history of type 2 diabetes, and there appears to be scant literature evaluating the importance of family history in the development of these metabolic changes. HIV disease alone has been associated with lipid abnormalities, although this may simply be a response to chronic infection. Plasma HDL-cholesterol decreases in early disease, followed by a further decline with advanced illness, accompanied by a rise in triglyceride and a reduction in LDL particle size, which has been suggested to be cytokine-mediated.

Protease inhibitors have been implicated in dyslipidaemia with increased plasma concentrations of total cholesterol and lipoprotein(a), usually with a decrease in HDL-cholesterol levels. Raised triglyceride levels appear most pronounced with ritonavir. The mechanism(s) for the metabolic effects of protease inhibitors remain to be determined; however, some interesting information is emerging from animal studies.[6] Ritonavir-treated mice have increased levels of the active cleaved form of the sterol regulatory element-binding protein (SREBP)-1c in liver cells, leading to increased activation of lipogenic genes.[7] Protease-inhibitor-mediated inhibition of protease activity preventing degradation of SREBP-1c, improved nutritional status or hyperinsulinaemia may further enhance this effect. Activation of SREBP-1c has also been implicated in the association of protease-inhibitor therapy, lipodystrophy and insulin resistance. It appears to modify the differentiation of pre-adipocytes to adipocytes. This led to hypoleptinaemia in mice, interestingly mimicking mouse models of congenital lipodystrophy with diabetes, hyperlipidaemia and hypoleptinaemia. Insulin resistance then leads to increased insulin production and hence downregulation of insulin receptor substrate. This further stimulates production of SREBP-1c in the liver and adipocytes, thereby generating a vicious cycle (reviewed in Mooser et al.[6]).

Treatment of these metabolic derangements remains problematic, particularly where excellent viraemic control must be balanced against adverse effects of the antiretroviral treatment.[8] Conservative measures such as exercise and low-fat diet, although not formally assessed in clinically controlled trials, are good preliminary measures. Management of hyperlipidaemia remains largely unresolved. Preliminary guidelines suggest a trial of diet plus exercise followed by fibrates or statins, dependent on the lipid profile. High-dose marine oils are useful in the treatment of severe hypertriglyceridaemia. Problems encountered include the already high prevalence of abnormal liver function tests, drug interactions particularly via cytochrome pathways and the increased risk of myalgia.

Given the association in mice between hypoleptinaemia and lipodystrophy, leptin may prove to be a useful adjunct to treatment in the future. It has been shown to improve both glycaemic control and to decrease triglyceride levels in patients with lipodystrophy and leptin deficiency.[9] In addition, in a small study, thiazolidinediones alone significantly improved insulin sensitivity and decreased total triglycerides, VLDL-cholesterol and total body fat.[10] The use of insulin combined with metformin and a glitazone, although not currently licensed in all countries, may prove a useful therapy in insulin-resistant patients.

References

1. Carr A, Cooper D. Adverse effects of antiretroviral therapy. *Lancet* 2000; **356**: 1423–30.

2. Carr A, Samaras K, Burton S et al. A syndrome of peripheral lipodystrophy, hyperlipidaemia and insulin resistance in patients receiving HIV protease inhibitors. *AIDS* 1998; **12**: F51–8.

3. Carr A, Samaras K, Thorisdottir A et al. Diagnosis, prediction and natural course of HIV-1 protease-inhibitor-associated lipodystrophy, hyperlipidaemia and diabetes mellitus: a cohort study. *Lancet* 1999; **353**: 2093–9.

4. Lomar A. Acute myocardial infarction in a 34-year-old HIV-positive female patient while undergoing antiretroviral therapy containing a protease inhibitor. *Braz J Infect Dis* 1999; **3**: 197–200.

5. Henry K. Severe premature coronary artery disease with protease inhibitors. *Lancet* 1998; **351**: 1328.

6. Mooser V, Carr A. Antiretroviral therapy-associated hyperlipidaemia in HIV disease. *Curr Opin Lipidol* 2001; **12**: 313–19.

7. Kuhel DJ, Woollett LA, Fichtenbaum CJ, Hui DY. HIV protease induced hyperlipidaemia and lipodystrophy is mediated through regulation of sterol regulatory element binding protein (SREBP) responsive genes. *Circulation* 2000; **102**(Suppl. II): II–360.

8. Dube PM, Sprecher D, Henry WK et al. Preliminary guidelines for the evaluation and management of dyslipidaemia in adults infected with human immunodeficiency virus and receiving antiretroviral therapy: recommendations of the Adult AIDS Clinical Trial Group Cardiovascular Disease focus group. *Clin Infect Dis* 2000; **31**: 1216–24.

9. Oral EA, Simha V, Ruiz E et al. Leptin-replacement therapy for lipodystrophy. *N Engl J Med* 2002; **346**: 570–8.

10. Walli R. Effects of troglitazone on insulin sensitivity in HIV-infected patients with protease inhibitor-associated diabetes mellitus. *Res Exp Med (Berl)* 2000; **199**: 253–62.

CASE 28: A CASE OF TYPE 2 DIABETES MELLITUS WITH MULTIPLE RISK FACTORS FOR IHD AND MULTIPLE COMPLICATIONS

Julia Ostberg and D John Betteridge

History

A 67-year-old woman with type 2 diabetes was reviewed in clinic. She had a history of hypercholesterolaemia, hypertension and ischaemic heart disease (IHD). She was an ex-smoker and had a family history of type 2 diabetes, hypercholesterolaemia and IHD (both parents died of myocardial infarctions, her father aged 51, her mother aged 68). She herself had 3-vessel coronary artery bypass grafts at the age of 56, but developed recurrent anginal symptoms 4 years later. Revascularization was not possible and she received medical management.

She was originally diagnosed as having type 2 diabetes aged 60, when she was found to have an elevated fasting plasma glucose and had an HbA1c of 11.6%. After her diagnosis of diabetes she was initially treated with diet, but quickly progressed to increasing doses of metformin, her body mass index (BMI) being 32, and finally to gliclazide as she remained poorly controlled. Table 1 shows how her diabetic and lipid control fluctuated with time and body mass index.

Heterozygous familial hypercholesterolaemia was diagnosed at the age of 49, when she was noted to have small xanthelasmata, as well as large xanthomata in the extensor tendons of her hands and Achilles tendons, the hallmark of familial hypercholesterolaemia. Statins had not yet been introduced at this time, and over the years she was treated with a combination of fibrates and anion-exchange resins. Her compliance with the latter was poor as she found them very inconvenient to take. She was switched to a statin once these became available

Table 1 Fluctuations in diabetic and lipid control with time and BMI

Age (years)	BMI (kg/m²)	HbA1c (%)	Total cholesterol (mmol/L)	LDL (mmol/L)	HDL (mmol/L)	TG (mmol/L)
49	33	–	16.2	–	–	3.8
60	32	11.6	6.3	4.2	1.1	2.1
65	26	7.5	4.6	2.6	1.2	1.7
67	30	8.5	5.9	3.8	1.2	2.0

and is currently taking atorvastatin 80 mg (maximum therapeutic dose). Table 1 shows her good response to statin treatment.

At her most recent clinic visit her blood pressure was well controlled at 123/62 mmHg, but glycaemic and lipid control was deteriorating (see Table 1). Peripheral neuropathy was diagnosed for the first time on objective testing. She was complaining of muscle aches, although her creatine kinase was only 101. In addition, she was taking metformin 3 g daily, gliclazide 240 mg daily, bisoprolol, valsartan, amlodipine, a nitrate, nicorandil, aspirin and hormone replacement therapy. She was strongly advised by the dietitian to try harder with her diet and to increase her exercise as far as possible (she had no regular exercise programme but her exercise tolerance was limited by her angina). She was advised to start insulin treatment with a single injection of Insulatard at night but she refused. It was agreed that she should increase her dose of gliclazide to the maximum recommended (320 mg daily) and make further effort with lifestyle changes, although insulin would probably be inevitable in the future. She was also advised to increase her intake of stanol ester-containing foods to improve her lipid profile.

Commentary and learning points

This case demonstrates the difficulties of managing an overweight patient who has multiple metabolic risk factors and complications. While this lady had been able to modify her lifestyle to some degree in that she gave up smoking and had achieved significant weight loss in the past, she was unable to maintain her momentum. The metabolic benefits of her weight loss are clearly seen, with improvement in both glycaemic and lipid control. She found it difficult to maintain her weight while taking a sulphonylurea, resulting in a deterioration of these parameters, and the introduction of insulin may compound the problem. Her exercise tolerance is limited by her anginal symptoms. She is in the vicious cycle seen so often in these patients – weight loss would improve control, but this is difficult to achieve in the presence of hypoglycaemic agents.

Our approach was to suggest bedtime Insulatard, titrated to achieve a pre-breakfast glucose level of 6–7 mmol/L, with continuation of metformin. This regimen has been shown to improve glycaemic control while minimizing weight gain.[1] Despite counselling, the patient refused insulin. Alternative options are limited. She was intolerant of acarbose.

Thiazolidenediones, which might reduce HbA1c by 1–1.5%, are not currently licensed for use as triple therapy and there are few trial data for this combination, although there are anecdotal reports of its use by physicians in the USA. The weight gain associated with this class of drug is of concern in an already obese patient, although the redistribution of adipose tissue may be beneficial.[2] In addition, the problem of fluid retention must be considered in a patient with ischaemic heart disease.

A weight-reducing drug could be considered, but the patient was intolerant of orlistat owing to its gastrointestinal side-effects, and sibutramine is contraindicated in patients with hypertension and ischaemic heart disease.

A comment should be made on the use of sulphonylurea drugs in patients with ischaemic heart disease. There has been much debate about whether sulphonylurea drugs worsen outcome in ischaemic heart disease by preventing cardiac preconditioning through inhibition of the K^+ ATP channels in the heart as well as in pancreatic beta-cells. To date, however, the evidence remains inconclusive.[3] This patient is also on nicorandil, a K^+ ATP channel opener, which has been found to have a protective effect in chronic stable angina[4] and there is evidence to suggest that there is no antagonism between nicorandil and sulphonylureas in terms of either angina or diabetes control.[5]

This patient has familial hypercholesterolaemia (FH) which has responded well to treatment with statins. It should be emphasized that severe hypercholesterolaemia is not a feature of diabetic dyslipidaemia, and other primary (FH in this case) and secondary causes such as hypothyroidism should be sought. Familial hypercholesterolaemia is characterized by mutations of the low density lipoprotein (LDL) receptor gene, leading to impaired LDL receptor activity and decreased removal of plasma LDL by the liver; plasma LDL-cholesterol concentrations in FH heterozygotes are typically double those of non-affected family members. Statins, by inhibiting the enzyme HMG-CoA reductase, the rate-determining step in cholesterol synthesis, up-regulate LDL receptor expression.[6]

The hypertriglyceridaemia in this case is not typical of FH and can be attributed to the metabolic syndrome. Addition of a fibrate might be considered, as this class of lipid-lowering drug particularly targets high triglyceride levels with low HDL levels,[7] but this would have to be done cautiously as combination therapy increases risk of side-effects, especially myositis. It is becoming clear, however, that the fibrate gemfibrozil is particularly implicated in interactions with statins. The patient currently complains of muscle aches despite a normal creatine kinase level. Incidence of musculoskeletal symptoms has been shown to differ little in patients on statins compared to placebo in large placebo-controlled trials.[8,9] Taking these considerations into account, it was decided to advise increased intake of plant sterols/stanol esters in the first instance. These can play an important role in management of hypercholesterolaemia.[10]

This patient's cardiovascular risk is greatly increased by her multiple metabolic pathologies. Heterozygous familial hypercholesterolaemia *per se* carries a high mortality rate, although this risk can be reduced with treatment.[11] In addition, she suffers from the metabolic syndrome with poorly controlled diabetes and hypercholesterolaemia. She manifested end-organ damage at an early age. Her management illustrates the difficulty for physicians of treating patients with multiple cardiovascular risk factors, and also the difficulty for patients of tolerating such polypharmacy in the context of already impaired quality of life.

References

1. Yki-Jarvinen H. Combination therapies with insulin in type 2 diabetes. *Diabetes Care* 2001; **24**: 758–67.

2. Schoonjans K, Auwerx J. Thiazolidenediones: an update. *Lancet* 2000; **355**: 1008–10.

3. Betteridge DJ, Close L. Diabetes, coronary heart disease and sulphonylureas – not the final word. *Eur Heart J* 2000; **21**: 790–2.

4. Gomma AH, Purcell HJ, Fox KM. Potassium channel openers in myocardial ischaemia: therapeutic potential of nicorandil. *Drugs* 2001; **61**: 1705–10.

5. Hata N, Takano M, Kunimi T, Kishida H, Takano T. Lack of antagonism between nicorandil and sulfonylurea in stable angina pectoris. *Int J Clin Pharmacol Res* 2001; **21**: 59–63.

6. Scriver CR, Beaudet AL, Valle D, Sly WS. *The Metabolic and Molecular Basis of Inherited Disease*, 8th edn. McGraw Hill Medical Publishing Division, 2001. Chapter 120.

7. Rubins HB, Robins SJ, Collins D *et al*. Gemfibrozil for the secondary prevention of coronary heart disease in men with low levels of high-density lipoprotein cholesterol. Veterans Affairs High-Density Lipoprotein Cholesterol Intervention Trial Study Group. *N Engl J Med* 1999; **341**: 410–18.

8. Pedersen TR, Berg K, Cook TJ *et al*. Safety and tolerability of cholesterol lowering with simvastatin during 5 years in the Scandinavian Simvastatin Survival Study. *Arch Intern Med* 1996; **156**: 2085–92.

9. MRC/BHF Heart Protection Study of cholesterol lowering with simvastatin in 20,536 high-risk individuals: a randomised placebo-controlled trial. *Lancet* 2002; **360**: 7–22.

10. Plat J, Kerckhoffs DA, Mensink RP. Therapeutic potential of plant sterols and stanols. *Curr Opin Lipidol* 2000; **11**: 571–6.

11. Scientific Steering Committee on behalf of the Simon Broome Register Group. Mortality in treated heterozygous familial hypercholesterolaemia: implications for clinical management. *Atherosclerosis* 1999; **142**: 105–112.

CASE 29: A POORLY CONTROLLED DIABETIC PATIENT WITH MANY COMPLICATIONS

Mehmooda Syeed, Sherri Blackstone and Serge Jabbour

History

Mr AL is a 52-year-old obese black male (5 feet 11 inches and 235 lb) with a past medical history of hypertension, who presented 12 years ago to his primary care physician for a routine follow-up visit. His hypertension was being treated with hydrochlorothiazide (HCTZ) 25 mg daily. Family history was noteworthy for type 2 diabetes mellitus in his mother and older sister and coronary artery disease in his father who experienced a myocardial infarction at the age of 52 years. Routine blood tests were carried out at which time his fasting blood glucose was 190 mg/dL.

On a subsequent follow-up visit, a random accucheck in the primary care physician's office revealed a blood glucose of 252. At that time, his blood pressure was 140/90 mm Hg. Further testing showed the patient to have a HbA1C of 9.5%, a urine microalbumin:creatinine ratio of 30 μg/mg, a total cholesterol of 220 mg/dL (HDL, 30; LDL, 140; triglycerides, 250 mg/dl) and a creatinine of 1.1 mg/dL. He underwent ophthalmological evaluation which revealed early changes of diabetic retinopathy.

Treatment and outcome

Mr AL was started on glipizide 5 mg twice a day and provided with a glucometer to measure his blood sugars at home. The aforementioned blood pressure was considered adequate and the patient continued on his current dose of HCTZ. Regarding his lipid management, the patient was instructed to reduce his fat intake and lose weight.

The patient was followed on a biannual basis for the next 5 years. His weight had progressively increased by 20 lb. Blood pressure remained around 150/90 mm Hg and fasting glucose readings at home averaged around 200. Glipizide was increased to 10 mg twice a day. His LDL increased to 160 mg/dL and at this point lovastatin 20 mg daily was added. The urinary microalbumin:creatinine ratio now increased to 70 μg/mg and the patient was prescribed lisinopril 10 mg daily. However, the patient was unable to tolerate this medication because of a chronic, non-productive cough.

Over time the patient also noted burning and numbness in his feet and started experiencing pain in his calves while walking, which was relieved at rest. Physical examination at this point was remarkable for markedly reduced popliteal and absent pedal pulses. In addition, Mr AL experienced some erectile dysfunction which was contributing to deteriorating marital relations. Although he felt frustrated by this issue, he was at the same time hesitant to mention this to his primary care physician and was never directly queried about the subject.

On one of his follow-up visits to his primary care physician, Mr AL mentioned that his activity had been further limited by occasional chest discomfort and exertional dyspnoea. A 12-lead EKG obtained in the office was found to be significant only for some non-specific ST-T wave changes and left ventricular hypertrophy. The patient was scheduled for an exercise stress test which had to be stopped secondary to severe bilateral lower extremity pains. A persantine thallium stress test was suggestive of anterolateral ischaemia, which was later confirmed by coronary angiography revealing multi-vessel coronary artery disease with predominant stenosis of his left anterior descending artery. Angioplasty with stent placement was performed and the patient was started on aspirin, lopressor and nitrates. Atorvastatin 20 mg daily was substituted for lovastatin. Metformin was added and maximized for better glycaemic control.

An arteriogram of the lower extremities showed significant femoral-popliteal atherosclerotic disease, right greater than left. Right femoral-popliteal bypass surgery was performed.

Over the subsequent years, the patient continued with worsening nephropathy and glycaemic control. Microalbuminuria progressed to 300 µg/mg and serum creatinine rose to 1.6 mg/dL. Metformin was discontinued and irbesartan was added for renoprotective effects and better blood pressure control. Rosiglitazone was added to the regimen, but later had to be discontinued because of excessive lower extremity oedema. Glipizide was stopped and the patient was started on a twice-daily insulin regimen. Around the same time, an ophthalmological examination was performed, and the patient was found to have background non-proliferative diabetic retinopathy. He continued with worsening neuropathy in both feet.

At age 51, Mr AL experienced an anterior wall myocardial infarction with subsequent left ventricular dysfunction and congestive heart failure. He underwent three-vessel coronary artery bypass graft (CABG) and pharmacological therapy was maximized. The patient was referred to an endocrinologist for intensive diabetes management.

In summary, Mr AL is an obese 52-year-old black male with a 12-year history of type 2 diabetes, hypertension and dyslipidaemia, who was inadequately managed over the years. He developed multiple end-organ complications, both microvascular and macrovascular, requiring not only pharmacological but also surgical intervention. His outlook has been altered immensely by these events.

Commentary

Type 2 diabetes mellitus is a rapidly increasing chronic and disabling disease which affects millions of individuals worldwide. The morbidity and mortality associated with this disease in the United States alone cost over US$100 billion per year. Whereas microvascular complications cause major disability, the macrovascular disease results in about 80% mortality as a result of cardiovascular endpoints. Effective and early treatment of patients can save many lives and billions of dollars every year.

Although there are no randomized trials demonstrating the benefits of early diagnosis through screening of asymptomatic individuals, there is sufficient indirect evidence to justify its use in high risk populations. For example, Mr AL was over 45 years of age, obese, hypertensive, had a strong family history of diabetes mellitus and belonged to a high-risk ethnic group (African–American).[1] A recent study conducted in over 3000 patients with impaired fasting and postprandial plasma glucose concentrations compared lifestyle modification (goal of 7% weight loss and at least 150 minutes of physical activity each week) with metformin therapy. The former showed a 58% reduction in the incidence of diabetes compared with 31% in the metformin group.[2] The HOPE (Heart Outcomes Prevention Evaluation) trial showed a 32% reduction in the risk of subsequent diabetes in association with ACE inhibition therapy.[3]

In our patient, a HbA1C of 9.5% and fasting blood glucose of around 200 mg/dL obviously reflected poor glycaemic control. A lack of symptoms may have been mistakenly perceived as adequate glycaemic control both by our patient and the health care provider, and led to very conservative therapy.

The optimal goal in type 2 diabetes therapy is to achieve a HbA1C of < 7%, fasting blood glucose between 80 and 120 and bedtime blood glucose between 100 and 140.[4] The UKPDS (UK Prospective Diabetes Study) has conclusively demonstrated a definite risk reduction in microvascular complications with improved glycaemic control. This prospective study included 3867 patients who were randomized into an intensively treated group (HbA1C 7.0%) compared with a conventionally treated group (HbA1C 7.9%), who were followed over a 10-year period. Compared with the conventional group, the intensive group showed a risk reduction of 12% for any diabetes-related endpoint, 10% risk reduction for any diabetes-related death and 6% for all-cause mortality. Most of the risk reduction was the result of a 25% risk reduction in microvascular endpoints. However, there was no significant difference in macrovascular complications between the two groups.[5]

Monotherapy is unlikely to achieve glycaemic goals in the majority of cases. Most monotherapies exhibit similar effects in improving HbA1c levels. However, those drugs that exclusively target postprandial hyperglycaemia (meglitinides, miglitol, acarbose) have less effective HbA1C-lowering effects than the other monotherapies.

Few studies have looked at initial therapy with combinations of oral antihyperglycaemic agents. Low dose glyburide/metformin in combination with lifestyle modification showed a 66% success in achieving a HbA1c of < 7%.[6] Similar results were shown in a study conducted in 83 patients with inadequately controlled type 2 diabetes. Subjects were randomized to continue with their pre-study metformin or a combination of metformin and repaglinide. Patients receiving combination therapy showed a HbA1C reduction from 8.3% to 6.9%. Overall, 59% of the patients in the combined therapy group achieved optimal glycaemic control with a HbA1C < 7.1%.[7]

There are various classes of oral antihyperglycaemic agents available for type 2 diabetes therapy and these agents have different mechanisms of action which can be additive. A rational approach would be to start therapy with a combination of drugs with different mechanisms of action and maximize their dosages as diabetes progresses.

The insulin resistance syndrome in type 2 diabetes causes an excessive rate of macrovascular complications. This syndrome is characterized by dyslipidaemia, central obesity, procoagulant state, endothelial dysfunction and abnormalities suggestive of a low-grade inflammatory state. Metformin and thiazolidinediones (TZDs) have been effective in improving the various components of the insulin resistance syndrome, whereas insulin secretagogues have been shown to have no effect.[8]

Diabetic patients often have a characteristic constellation of dyslipidaemia, including elevated triglycerides, reduced HDL, small dense LDL and borderline to high LDL cholesterol levels. This profile is termed atherogenic or diabetic dyslipidaemia.[8] For all adults with diabetes, regardless of the presence of known cardiovascular disease, the primary treatment goal is to achieve an LDL cholesterol of < 100 mg/dL. Studies have shown striking reductions in coronary events in both primary and secondary prevention trials. The Cholesterol and Recurrent Events (CARE) trial and the Scandinavian Simvastatin Survival Study (4S) demonstrated that aggressive LDL cholesterol lowering with statins (pravastatin in CARE and simvastatin in 4S) significantly reduces the risk of recurrent myocardial infarctions, cardiovascular death, strokes and the need for revascularization procedures.[9,10] The Atorvastatin Versus Revascularization Treatment Study (AVERT) found that aggressive LDL cholesterol reduction with atorvastatin was more effective in reducing ischaemic events than coronary angioplasty.[11]

The prevalence of hypertension in type 2 diabetes is higher than in the general population. It is associated with an increased rate of microvascular complications and also increases the already high risk of coronary artery disease associated with type 2 diabetes.[12] The primary goal of therapy is to decrease blood pressure to < 130/80 mm Hg in diabetics. However, a more aggressive goal of < 125/75 mm Hg is needed for patients with renal insufficiency or with proteinuria > 1 g/day.[13] A recent review which analysed the use of ACE inhibitors in various clinical trials has demonstrated significant benefit from ACE inhibitors compared with other therapies in reducing acute myocardial infarction, cardiovascular mortality, or all-cause mortality as endpoints. Such results were not seen in the UKPDS.[14]

Diabetic nephropathy is the leading cause of end-stage renal disease (ESRD) in the United States. In most cases, ESRD from diabetic nephropathy can be preventable. Microalbuminuria by itself and its rate of progression are not only a risk factor for renal failure but also a strong predictor of cardiovascular morbidity and mortality.[15] The major risk factors for development of diabetic nephropathy are poor glycaemic control and coexistent hypertension. Although the renoprotective effects of ACE inhibitors are well established in type 1 diabetes, there are no similar studies published addressing similar effects in type 2 diabetes. A recent study with angiotensin-2-receptor blockers (ARBs) showed this class of agents to be effective in protecting against the progression of nephropathy in type 2 diabetics. Of note, their effect was found to be independent of the blood pressure reduction.[16]

A meta-analysis of 16 prospective cohort studies has shown the relative risk of death from coronary artery disease in diabetic patients to be 2.58 in women and 1.85 in men.[17] Studies in the past have shown the association of diabetes mellitus with higher rates of restenosis post-angioplasty. The BARI trial (Bypass Angioplasty Revascularization Investigation) compared CABG versus angioplasty in diabetics with coronary ischaemia. This trial showed definite superiority of patients who underwent CABG (19% deaths in CABG versus 34% in angioplasty). These results support CABG as the preferred procedure for initial revascularization among diabetics with multi-vessel coronary artery disease.[18] The Heart Outcomes Prevention Evaluation (HOPE) is a recent landmark trial which studied 3577 patients at high risk for subsequent vascular events. The patients were randomized to receive ramipril, vitamin E, both, or neither. Ramipril-treated patients experienced a 25% relative risk reduction of the primary composite endpoints (myocardial infarction, stroke, cardiovascular death).[3]

In summary, diabetes mellitus is an enormous burden on the health care system in terms of both financial and psychophysiological costs. The challenge for primary care physicians and endocrinologists is to screen high-risk patients, provide strict glycaemic and blood pressure control, and achieve aggressive LDL cholesterol reduction. There should be annual screening for microvascular complications, including microalbuminuria, which is a risk factor for progressive nephropathy and cardiovascular mortality. As previously discussed, diabetes mellitus is considered an inflammatory syndrome, and strict adherence to glycaemic, blood pressure and lipid goals should provide control and prevent or delay complications from this endemic disease.

131

References

1. American Diabetes Association, Screening for type 2 diabetes. *Diabetes Care* 2001; 24 (Suppl 1): S21–S24.

2. Diabetes Prevention Program Research Group. Reduction in the incidence of type 2 diabetes with lifestyle intervention or metformin. *N Engl J Med* 2002; 346: 393–403.

3. The Heart Outcomes Prevention Evaluation Study Investigators. Effects of angiotensin converting-enzyme inhibitor, ramipril, on cardiovascular events in high-risk patients. *N Engl J Med* 2000; 342: 145–53.

4. American Diabetes Association. Standards of medical care for patients with diabetes mellitus. *Diabetes Care* 2000; 23 (Suppl 1): S32–S42.

5. UK Prospective Diabetes Study Group. Intensive blood glucose control with sulphonylureas or insulin compared with conventional treatment and risk of complications in patients with type 2 diabetes (UKPDS 33). *Lancet* 1998; 352: 837–53.

6. Davidson J, Garber A, Mooradian A et al. Metformin/glyburide tablets as first-line treatment in type 2 diabetes: distribution of HbA1c response (abstract). *Diabetes* 2000; 49 (Suppl 1): 1494.

7. Moses R, Carter J, Slobodniuk R et al. Effect of repaglinide addition to metformin monotherapy on glycemic control in patients with type 2 diabetes. *Diabetes Care* 1999; 22: 119–24.

8. O'Keefe JH, Miles JM, Harris WH et al. Improving the adverse cardiovascular prognosis of type 2 diabetes. *Mayo Clin Proc* 1999; 74: 171–80.

9. Sacks FM, Pfeffer MA, Moye LA et al. The effect of pravastatin on coronary events after myocardial infarction in patients with average cholesterol levels. *N Engl J Med* 1996; 335: 1001 9.

10. Randomised trial of cholesterol lowering in 4444 patients with coronary heart disease: the Scandinavian Simvastatin Survival Study (4S). *Lancet* 1994; 344: 1383–9.

11. Pitt B, Waters D, Brown WV et al. Aggressive lipid lowering therapy compared with angioplasty in stable coronary artery disease. *N Engl J Med* 1999; 341: 70–6.

12. UK Prospective Diabetes Study Group (UKPDS 23). Risk factors for coronary artery disease in non-insulin-dependent diabetes mellitus. *BMJ* 1998; 316: 823–8.

13. Elliott WJ, Weir DR, Black HR. Cost-effectiveness of the lower treatment goal (JNC VI) for diabetic hypertensive patients: Joint National Committee on Prevention, Detection, Evaluation, and Treatment of High Blood Pressure. *Arch Intern Med* 2000; 169: 1277–83.

14. Pahor M, Psaty BM, Alderman MH et al. Therapeutic benefits of ACE inhibitors and other antihypertensive drugs in patients with type 2 diabetes. *Diabetes Care* 2000; 23: 888–92.

15. Spoelstra-De Man A, Brouwer CB, Stehouwer CDA et al. Rapid progression of albumin excretion is an independent predictor of cardiovascular mortality in patients with type 2 diabetes and microalbuminuria. *Diabetes Care* 2001; **24**: 2097–101.

16. Parving HH, Lehnert H, Brochner-Mortensen J et al. The effect of irbesartan on the development of diabetic nephropathy in patients with type diabetes. *N Engl J Med* 2001; **345**: 870–8.

17. Lee WL, Cheung AM, Cape D et al. Impact of diabetes on coronary artery disease in women and men. A meta-analysis of prospective studies. *Diabetes Care* 2000; **23**: 962–8.

18. Schaff HV, Rosen AD, Shemin RJ et al. Clinical and operative characteristics of patients randomized to coronary artery bypass surgery in the bypass angioplasty revascularization investigation (BARI). *Am J Cardiol* 1995; **75**: 180–260.

CASE 30: ATYPICAL CHEST PAIN IN A YOUNG DIABETIC WOMAN: THE VALUE OF MEDIA EDUCATION

Graham Jackson

History

A 37-year-old lady complained of an ache in the chest of 6 weeks' duration. She felt it was 'bad heartburn' but she had also noticed a numbness affecting her left arm. She had read an article on heart disease in women and had become concerned about the numbness after reading of its association with coronary disease. Of concern was the relationship of the numb sensation to exertion and in particular, inclines or climbing stairs. On direct questioning she admitted to being a little short of breath with a tight sensation in the chest, again brought on by effort but also promptly relieved by rest. The pain had woken her on one occasion.

She has been an insulin-dependent diabetic for 18 years, has never smoked and a recent random cholesterol was 5.7 mm/L. Married with two young children (aged 5 and 8 years) she normally had an active lifestyle.

Examination and investigations

On examination she was slim and anxious. Her blood pressure was 150/80 mmHg and her pulse, heart sounds and lung fields were normal. A resting 12-lead ECG was normal.

Opinion

The GP thought the pain was musculoskeletal but because of her diabetes stated '... Clearly cardiac ischaemia is a possibility'. I felt she was describing angina pectoris but expressed my surprise in correspondence. I was worried about the pain that woke her.

Treatment and outcome

I commenced her on diltiazem because she admitted to occasional hypoglycaemic attacks and I was afraid these might be masked by beta-blockade. Aspirin 75 mg daily was introduced.

Given her young age and presentation I performed an urgent coronary angiogram which identified a single critical left anterior descending stenosis and normal left ventricular function (Figure 1). Using the direct stent technique the lesion was successfully dilated to leave no residual stenosis (Figure 2a and b).

Her cholesterol fasting was 4.61 mmol/L, HDL 1.7, LDL 2.54 and triglycerides 0.81 mmol/L. Her C-reactive protein, lipoprotein (a) and homocysteine were normal. I commenced her on pravastatin 40 mg daily, given that she had developed coronary disease at an early age with the important risk factor of diabetes, following the philosophy that whatever the cholesterol at the onset of coronary disease it is too high for the individual. Statins also have additional properties to lipid lowering which benefit endothelial function.

She returned to a symptom-free active life. On pravastatin her cholesterol fell to 3.2 mmol/L (HDL 1.46, LDL 1.44, triglycerides 0.65). Her blood pressure remained raised but reached the target of 130–135 mmHg systolic following the introduction of an ACE inhibitor, chosen because of the strong evidence base of benefit in diabetics.

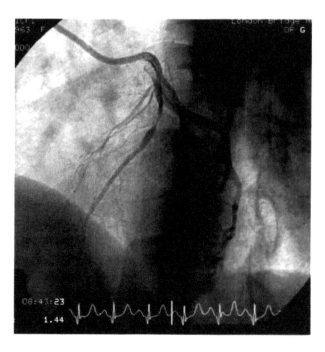

Figure 1 *Coronary angiogram demonstrating a critical left anterior descending stenosis.*

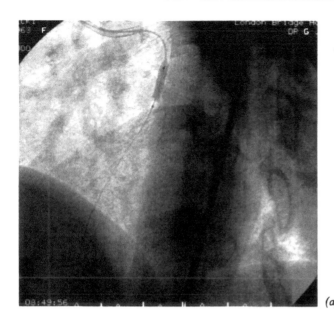

Figure 2 *(a) Stent in position for deployment. (b) Angiographic result.*

(a)

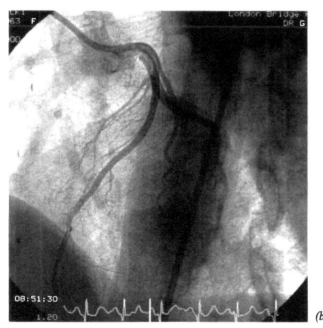

(b)

Learning points

- Coronary disease is common in women but may present atypically.
- Premenopausal women are an increasing management challenge. Gender bias needs to be eliminated.

- Diabetics with no known coronary disease have the same cardiac risk as non-diabetics who already have vascular disease.
- All diabetics at diagnosis should be considered for prophylactic statin and ACE inhibitor/angiotension II therapy.

CASE 31: BLOOD PRESSURE WITH COMPLICATIONS

Per L Poulsen, Klavs W Hansen and
Carl E Mogensen

History

A 41-year-old man was admitted to our hospital with a foot ulcer. For the previous 3–4 months he had complained of a feeling of 'walking on cotton wool' and discrete polyuria and polydipsia, but otherwise he had felt well. He was formerly in good health and had no familial predisposition to endocrinological diseases.

Examination and investigations

Blood pressure was 160/115 mmHg, heart rate 86 bpm, body temperature 37.8°C. BMI was 33 kg/m². A severely infected deep plantar ulceration was present on the right foot. The foot was warm with bounding pulses. Deep tendon reflexes could not be elicited and biothesiometry showed total loss of vibration sense. X-rays of the right foot demonstrated osteomyelitis. Eye examination and subsequent fundus photography revealed proliferative retinopathy and hard exudates.

Blood values were as follows: blood glucose, 18 mmol/L; WBC, 19.3 10⁹/L; C-reactive protein, 3000 nmol/L; pNa^+, 139 mmol/L; $p\text{-}K^+$, 4.5 mmol/L; $p\text{-}HCO_3$, 18 mmol/L; p-urea, 3.8 mmol/L; arterial pH, 7.37; cholesterol, 5.7 mmol/L; (HDL, 1.1 mmol/L; LDL, 3.8 mmol/L). Moderate ketonuria was present, there was no proteinuria. Urinary albumin: creatinine ratio was 15 mg/mmol (< 2.5 mg/mmol).

Diagnosis

Newly diagnosed type 2 diabetes with multiple complications.

Treatment and outcome

Broad-spectrum antibiotics were initiated, and collections of pus were drained in several surgical procedures over the next 2 months of hospitalization. Digiti IV and V had to be amputated but eventually the patient maintained walking capability. Insulin treatment was started. He was treated with retinal laser photocoagulation with only discretely reduced visual accuracy. There were no signs of angina pectoris and a coronary angiogram showed no stenosis. Hyperlipidaemia was treated with a statin. Due to incipient nephropathy with microalbuminuria and high BP (measured in the supine situation because of the foot ulcer), antihypertensive treatment with ACE inhibitor, beta-blocker and diuretics was initiated. After discharge from the hospital he was seen in our outpatients clinic where he complained about dizziness, especially in the upright position. Blood pressure was 75/50 mmHg in the standing position; 24-h ambulatory blood pressure measurement demonstrated (Figure 1) reversed circadian blood pressure rhythm. The antihypertensive treatment was changed to primarily administration at bedtime, and subsequently daytime BP increased and the dizziness disappeared. Autonomic function was assessed by classical cardiovascular reflex tests demonstrating almost no inspiratory-expiratory difference (2.95 bmp) and severe orthostatic hypotension (systolic BP drop of 40 mmHg). In addition, power spectral analysis of heart rate variability (HRV) was performed. This technique, which is also designated frequency domain

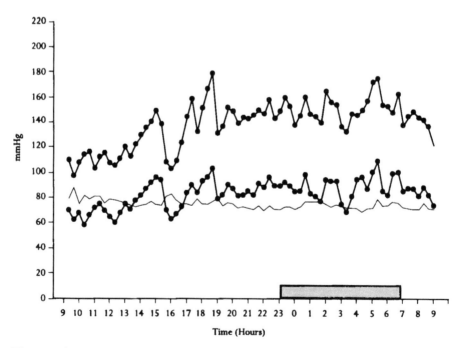

Figure 1 Reversed circadian blood pressure rhythm as demonstrated by 24-h ambulatory blood pressure measurement: 24-h BP, 137/83 mmHg; daytime BP, 134/81 mmHg; night-time BP, 151/89 mmHg.

analysis, decomposes the total RR interval variability and identifies systematic oscillations according to predominant wavelengths. Two major components with different frequency bands can be identified by power spectral analysis of HRV. The respiratory-dependent high frequency oscillations are mediated purely by vagal activity, whereas the low frequency oscillations in the upright position are mediated by interaction of sympathetic and vagal activity. Outpatient demonstrated severely reduced HRV in both the high and the low frequency components. Erectile dysfunction was treated with sildenafil.

Commentary

Type 2 diabetes is present in a subclinical form long before diagnosis and late complications are not unusual at diagnosis. Outpatient presented with neuropathy (both peripheral and autonomic), retinopathy and incipient nephropathy. The association between diabetic autonomic neuropathy and disturbed circadian variation of BP is well described, as is the association between diabetic nephropathy and attenuated circadian BP variation. High nocturnal BP may have prognostic implications. In a study in type 2 diabetic patients Nakano et al[1] reported that reversed circadian BP rhythm was associated with significantly increased incidence of both fatal and non-fatal vascular events. In patients with essential systolic hypertension, Staessen et al[2] reported that systolic night-time BP predicted cardiovascular endpoints better than daytime level in the placebo group, and cardiovascular risk increased significantly with increasing night/day ratio, also after adjustment for 24-h BP and other risk factors.

What did I learn from this case?

Autonomic neuropathy is an often forgotten complication in diabetes. In the presence of this complication, measurement of 24-h ambulatory may reveal daytime hypotension and nocturnal hypertension – changes that are important to recognize from a therapeutic point of view.

How much did this case alter my approach to the care and treatment of my patients with diabetes?

Patients with type 2 diabetes should be screened for late complications right from the time of diagnosis. In patients with autonomic neuropathy we perform 24-h ambulatory in order to assess BP more precisely and to tailor antihypertensive treatment in a rational way.

141

Further reading

Hansen KW, Poulsen PL, Ebbehøj E. Blood pressure elevation in diabetes: results from 24-h ambulatory blood pressure recordings. In: Mogensen CE, ed. *The Kidney and Hypertension in Diabetes Mellitus*. Boston: Kluwer Academic Publishers, 2000: 339–62.

Hournung RS, Mahler RF, Raftery EB. Ambulatory blood pressure and heart rate in diabetic patients: an assessment of autonomic function. *Diabetic Med* 1989; 6: 579–85.

Mølgaard H, Christensen PD, Hermansen K, Sørensen KE, Christensen CK, Mogensen CE. Early recognition of autonomic dysfunction in microalbuminuria: significance for cardiovascular mortality in diabetes mellitus? *Diabetologia* 1994; 37: 788–96.

Poulsen PL, Ebbehøj E, Hansen KW, Mogensen CE. 24-h blood pressure and autonomic function is related to albumin excretion within the normoalbuminuric range in IDDM patients. *Diabetologia* 1997; 40: 718–25.

References

1. Nakano S, Fukuda M, Hotta F et al. Reversed circadian blood pressure rhythm is associated with occurrences of both fatal and nonfatal vascular events in NIDDM subjects. *Diabetes* 1998; 47: 1501–6.

2. Staessen JA, Thijs L, Fagard R et al. Predicting cardiovascular risk using conventional vs ambulatory blood pressure in older patients with systolic hypertension. Systolic Hypertension in Europe Trial Investigators. *JAMA* 1999; 282: 539–46.

CASE 32: A TOUCH OF DIABETES

Merlin Thomas and Mark Cooper

History

A 68-year-old man is admitted to his local hospital with a shortness of breath. He has felt this way for some weeks but over the last few days has become increasingly breathless. He denies any chest pain or palpitations, claiming to have been fit and well until the last few months. He suggests that 'just a touch of diabetes' is his only problem.

His first contact with hospital had been 8 years previously, when he was referred for urological investigation. The referral letter described the patient complaining of nocturia and impotence. Rectal examination revealed an enlarged smooth prostate. His blood pressure at this clinical visit was noted to be elevated at 170/90 mmHg.

He presented for elective transurethral surgery 6 months later. On the day of the operation he was reviewed by an anaesthetist, who noted him as being a 'short round man' weighing 104 kg and measuring 165 cm in height. His blood pressure was 155/90 mmHg. The remainder of his clinical examination was noted to be unremarkable. Pre-operative blood tests showed albumin 36 g/L, urea 9.2 mmol/L, creatinine 120 (hospital laboratory normal range 50–120 µmol/L). A ward urinalysis on the morning of surgery was positive for protein and glucose.

Following the operation he was referred back to his general practitioner (GP) for further investigations. His blood pressure was elevated at 180/90 mmHg with no orthostatic change. The GP noted blood and protein in his urine following his surgery. Random capillary testing confirmed an elevated blood glucose at a level of 9.2 mmol/L. At this time he was informed he had 'a touch of diabetes' and instructed to lose weight, improve his diet and exercise more often. He was commenced on atenolol 50 mg a day for his blood pressure. At follow-up visits his systolic blood pressure remained around 145–155 mmHg and bendrofluazide 2.5 mg/day was added. Following the prescribed diet and exercise regime, he lost 6 kg over the next year. His blood glucose measurements were between 6 and 9 mmol/L every time he saw his GP, although his HbA1c remained elevated at 9%. He then moved away, presenting again only before his hospital admission with shortness of breath.

Examination and investigations

Examination at the time of his admission reveals an obese man weighing 115 kg. His blood pressure is 165/85 and blood sugar 13.6 mmol/L. He is clinically in biventricular failure with pitting oedema and bilateral lung crepitations with a left-sided pleural effusion. An electrocardiogram demonstrates atrial fibrillation with T wave inversion across the anterior leads with inferior Q waves without acute ST changes. An echocardiogram confirms his poor cardiac function with inferior akinesis and significant left ventricular hypertrophy. He has reduced sensation to pinprick and light touch over his lower limbs. He has a left femoral bruit and absent pedal pulses. Fundoscopy shows grade II hypertensive changes with a number of soft exudates.

His creatinine is now 250 μmol/L with a urea of 19 mmol/L. His potassium is 5.5 mmol/L. Urinalysis shows '++' proteinuria. His blood haemoglobin A1c is 8.3%. His total cholesterol is elevated at 7.8 mmol/L (LDL cholesterol, 153 mg/dL (4.0 mmol/L); HDL cholesterol, 36 mg/dL (0.93 mmol/L); triglyceride level, 350 mg/dL (4.0 mmol/L); HDL/total cholesterol ratio 0.12).

He is commenced on loop diuretic and digitalized. Four days later, he is feeling much better. An angiogram is performed, which shows diffuse atherosclerotic disease of both the left anterior descending and right coronary arteries with multiple stenoses and an occluded dominant circumflex artery.

He is discharged the following day and instructed to return in 1 week's time. At this clinic visit he continues to feel well, although a blood test taken the previous day shows that his creatinine has now risen to 350 μmol/L and his potassium remains elevated at 5.7 mmol/L. He is referred urgently to a nephrologist. 'Am I going to need dialysis?' the man asks.

Commentary

There seems little doubt that cases such as this will become increasingly common in adult medicine. More than 11 million Americans have both diabetes and hypertension. Many of these already have or will develop renal and cardiovascular damage.[1]

An early diagnosis forms the cornerstone upon which the current management of diabetic complications rests. Many of the interventions discussed in this book are more efficacious the earlier they are initiated, particularly before overt disease becomes established. Identification of patients with early renal disease can only be achieved by regular screening for microalbuminuria in patients with NIDDM, vascular disease and hypertension from their time of diagnosis. International guidelines on the management of NIDDM reflect this fact, although there are no controlled trials to confirm that screening slows progression of proteinuria.[2] While screening may offer the potential for early intervention, many patients with

NIDDM remain asymptomatic and present late with irreversibly impaired renal and cardiac function. In the AUSDIAB study, $> 8\%$ of patients with undiagnosed type 2 diabetes had proteinuria and over 6% had renal impairment (GFR $< 65 \text{ mL/min}/1.73 \text{ m}^2$) (AUSDIAB study, personal communication).[3] This figure may be even greater in some communities, where there is a lack of availability or delayed acceptance of medical care.[3] At least in these high-risk groups, it is possible that the pre-emptive rise of agents that block the renin angiotensin system (RAs) in all patients with NIDDM may ultimately be more cost-effective than screening for signs of established renal injury.[4]

Myocardial ischaemic may also be silent and progressive in diabetes, reflecting autonomic neuropathy, accelerated coronary atherosclerosis and an increase in vascular events in general (both silent and symptomatic).[5] Early identification of risk factors for cardiovascular events (such as proteinuria, hypertension, hyperlipidaemia, renal impairment, etc.) is potentially more important, as the main cause of mortality in patients with overt nephropathy is overwhelmingly cardiovascular.[1] The role of additional screening for silent ischaemia is controversial.[6] The diagnosis of unrecognized coronary artery disease clearly reinforces aggressive management of risk factors. However, screening in high-risk individuals has the potential to identify patients who may benefit from re-vascularization.

Accurate estimation of renal function is an important part of the management of patients with overt nephropathy. An isolated serum creatinine concentration should not be used as the sole indicator of renal function, particularly when evaluating creatinine measurements in the context of so-called 'normal concentration ranges'.[7] Substantial damage can occur with very little change in serum creatinine as a result of compensatory hyperfiltration in remaining nephrons. Clearance estimated from urinary creatinine collections may also prove inaccurate owing to incomplete urine collection and overestimation of the glomerular filtration rate (GFR) at low levels of renal function (due to increased tubular secretion of creatinine). This can only be partly corrected using an average of urea and creatinine clearance.[8] A calculated GFR (using formulae such as employed in the Modification of Diet in Renal Disease (MDRD) Study[9] or the Cockroft–Gault) with correction for body surface area allows a better estimation of renal function. However, such formulae may still be insensitive to early damage and inaccurate at extremes of body mass. In our case, both the Cockroft–Gault (55 mL/min) and the extended MDRD formula (53 mL/min), would have documented renal impairment at the time of the first presentation. Along with the presence of proteinuria, this should have identified this patient as being at significant risk of progressive renal disease.

A number of interventions in NIDDM has been shown to prevent the onset of proteinuria and slow the transition from microalbuminuria to overt albuminuria. But what about patients with NIDDM and overt diabetic nephropathy? By the time the serum creatinine is 150 μmol/L are renal structural changes too advanced to benefit from intervention? Is the damage already done?

Blood pressure control appears to be the most important intervention in type 2 diabetes. Up to 85% of patients with NIDDM and overt nephropathy also have hypertension.[10] Elevated systolic and diastolic BP accelerates the progression of diabetic nephropathy to end-stage renal disease (ESRD) and the rate of decline in renal function in a number of studies closely correlates with blood pressure levels achieved.[9,11] Clinical studies of both diabetic and non-diabetic renal disease have shown that blood pressure control can retard the progression of renal failure.[1,12] For some time, international guidelines for the management of patients with NIDDM and proteinuria have encouraged blood pressure targets (< 125/75 mmHg) below even those set for patients with occult disease (< 135/80 mmHg).[13,14] However, it has been only very recently that studies have confirmed the importance of aggressive blood pressure control in patients with advanced NIDDM and proteinuria to prevent progression to ESRD.[15,16]

These is also evidence that reductions in proteinuria (over and above blood pressure control) in patients with diabetes and renal impairment correlate with reductions in renal disease progression.[1,17–19] Specific therapies that target reductions in proteinuria might therefore be expected to confer more renoprotection than other agents in patients with overt nephropathy. Initially, a number of studies failed to show any favourable effect of ACE inhibitors in NIDDM with overt nephropathy either in terms of reduction of proteinuria or progression to ESRD. In particular, two studies in patients with type 2 diabetes with overt nephropathy[20,21] concluded that ACE inhibitors may not affect GFR reduction rate beyond their antihypertensive effect. The HOT[22] and UKPDS[11] studies also suggested that optimal blood pressure control (however it is achieved) may be beneficial. On the other hand, the CAPPP study showed that ACE inhibitors were superior to treatment based on diuretics and beta-blockers.[23] In a small randomized study of 30 patients with type 2 diabetes and overt nephropathy, urine protein dropped significantly only in the ACE inhibitor-treated group (4.4 to 0.56 g/day) and creatinine clearance decreased only in the nifedipine group.[24] Subsequent evidence (including the meta-analysis of Weidmann et al[25] now strongly suggests that GFR is better preserved in ACE inhibitor-treated patients with overt nephropathy than in those treated with beta-blockers, diuretics or nifedipine.

Recent evidence also suggests that hypertensive patients with overt nephropathy may further benefit from therapy with angiotensin receptor blockers (ARBs). Two recent large trials[15,16] suggest that ARBs may exert significant renoprotective effects in late stage nephropathy, reducing progression to renal failure by about a third, over and above the effects of blood pressure reduction alone. In addition, ARBs may be better tolerated than ACE inhibitors, with fewer side-effects (particularly cough). Although there have been no large studies comparing ARB and ACE inhibitors on renal function in type 2 diabetes, at least theoretically, drugs that interrupt the renin angiotensin system (RAS) should offer, at least theoretically, a similar degree of renoprotection.[26]

146

In practice, most patients, and particularly those with established nephropathy and renal impairment, will require multiple agents to achieve blood pressure goals, particularly those with established nephropathy and renal impairment. Clinical trials that have randomized patients to lower levels of BP require an average range of 2.8–4.2 different antihypertensive agents to achieve desired targets.[1] The combination of an ACE inhibitor and ARBs may result in greater renoprotection and blood pressure reductions than either agent used alone (CALM Study Group: M Copper, personal communication)[28] but has yet to be submitted to large trials. The combination of ACE inhibitor in conjunction with long-acting calcium channel blockers (CCBs) may have additional beneficial effects, particularly in terms of proteinuria and vascular events.[27,28] Diuretics may also be a useful adjunct, to potentiate the blood pressure-lowering effects of ACE inhibitors and ARBs without adverse effects on glucose homeostasis.

Another important intervention in patients with overt nephropathy may be maintaining lifestyle changes and dietary changes particularly with regard to weight loss in obese patients. As seen in this case, success can be short-lived with remission and weight gain the corollary of loss of vigilance. In patients with obesity, weight reduction reduces cardiovascular risk and improves metabolic control.[29] Improvements in blood pressure control following weight reduction should slow the progression of renal disease. In addition, there is some evidence that obesity may contribute to hyperfiltration and progressive nephrectomy, Praga et al.[31] found that among 14 obese (BMI $> 30 \, \text{kg/m}^2$) patients, 13 (92%) developed proteinuria/renal insufficiency. In contrast, among 59 patients with BMI $< 30 \, \text{kg/m}^2$, only 7 (12%) developed these complications. Currently, there is insufficient evidence to show that weight loss in obese patients per se can slow the progression of renal disease. In addition, some recent studies suggest that a higher BMI may be associated with increased survival at ESRD.[32] Care must be observed so as not to confuse therapeutic weight loss with catabolism on account of uraemia or weight gain because of fluid retention.

It is also controversial whether aggressive glycaemic control is valuable once a patient has developed overt nephropathy. Aggressive management of hypertension is clearly more important than glycaemic control in reducing cardiovascular events and slowing renal disease progression. However, in patients achieving blood pressure targets, does control of blood glucose confer any additional benefit? Certainly hyperglycaemia risks dehydration in the acute setting and, in the long term, has effects on cardiac function and renal perfusion. Some studies have suggested that poor glycaemic control can accelerate the loss of renal function in diabetic nephropathy.[33] However, large studies have failed to show any evidence that strict glycaemic control per se retards renal progression once overt nephropathy is present.[34] In addition, as renal function fails, tight glycaemic control becomes more hazardous with an increased risk of hypoglycaemia. Rising insulin levels may also act to increase blood pressure.[35] As there is sufficient evidence that glycaemic control may reduce both macrovascular events and microvascular complications of diabetes, it is reasonable to suggest that optimization of metabolic control remains worthwhile.

Hyperkalaemia is also a significant problem in diabetic nephropathy, related to renal impairment as well as associated hyporeninaemic hypoaldosteronism. The risk of hyperkalaemia is further increased with the use of ACE inhibitors or ARBs. In most studies using ARBs in advanced renal failure the incidence of hyperkalaemia is < 10%,[15,16,18] although some studies have documented the risk of hyperkalaemia with ACE inhibitor treatment in > 50% of patients.[36] It is important to note that both beta-blockers and digoxin may also contribute to the hyperkalaemia seen in our case, although the use of potassium-sparing diuretics in combination with an ACE inhibitor may be more dangerous.[37] NSAIDs and COX-2 inhibitors may also predispose to life-threatening hyperkalaemia in patients with renal impairment.[38]

Clinicians often use the issue of hyperkalaemia as an important reason to avoid renoprotective therapy with an ACE inhibitor or ARB. Yet it is precisely in cases like the one described, that ACE inhibition would seem most valuable. Although hyperkalaemia is common, the degree of hyperkalaemia seen in cases like this is seldom severe or life-threatening. Once the acute effects of contrast toxicity and reductions in intravascular volume in our patient have resolved, the cautious introduction of a low dose of an ACE inhibitor (or ARB) may yet be both possible and beneficial. The majority of patients with hyperkalaemia can be managed with the institution of a low-potassium diet or the addition of a diuretic agent. However, it is important to remember, as in this case, that thiazine diuretics are not effective with advanced renal insufficiency.

Correction of any reversible factors that contribute to a decreased GFR can restore a level of renal function compatible with a more conservative approach to care and defer the need for dialysis. In particular, pre-existing renal impairment is a major risk factor for the development of radiocontrast-induced acute tubular necrosis (CN). The incidence of a rise in the plasma creatinine concentration of > 50% above baseline or > 88 μmol/L is 4–11% with mild to moderate renal insufficiency alone.[39–42] This risk is increased to > 40% by more advanced renal dysfunction, heart failure, and concurrent administration of nephrotoxic drugs or volume depletion. It is controversial whether diabetes *per se* represents an independent risk for CN. A number of prospective studies have suggested that patients with diabetes and normal renal function have a similar incidence of CN to patients without diabetes. There is little doubt, however, that the combination of diabetes and renal impairment significantly increases the risk of renal injury and the requirement for dialysis. Although this injury is usually reversible, in patients with diabetes, baseline renal function may not be restored in patients with diabetes.[43]

Where possible, patients with diabetes and renal impairment should avoid the use of imaging studies that involve contrast and, in particular, multiple studies performed in rapid succession. A particularly challenging time is during the investigation and management of acute pulmonary oedema. Volume depletion can increase renal vasoconstriction and augment contrast toxicity, although it clearly forms an important part of heart failure management. Where intravenous contrast forms an indispensable tool to management, low-osmolality, non-ionic or gadolinium-based contrast media may be less nephrotoxic in patients with renal failure.[40,44] Lower contrast doses may also be less nephrotoxic.[45] Other interventions may also be beneficial, including pre-hydration with saline (although this may be impractical in patients with significant CHF). Forced diuresis and vasodilators appear to confer no additional advantage and may be harmful to patients with diabetes. N-Acetylcysteine, a thiol-containing antioxidant, shows promise for protection against contrast-induced nephropathy.[46]

So will this patient require dialysis? If his current rate of decline in renal function were to continue (~5 mL/min per year) he would reach a level of renal function requiring dialysis in 2–3 years. Additional renal insults (such as drug toxicity, dehydration, contrast, etc.) may hasten this progression, while aggressive treatment of his blood pressure with an agent that interrupts the RAS may provide him with (on average) an additional 6 12 months without dialysis.[17] However, his chances of surviving to ESRD are not good. In a man with diabetes, renal impairment and diffuse atherosclerosis in his coronary as well as peripheral vasculature, there is a 50% risk of a cardiovascular event in the next 5 years.[47] His chances of surviving such an event are also impaired.

Like silent myocardial ischaemia, it is important to recognize silent renal disease in NIDDM and treat early. While early intervention is the cornerstone of the management of diabetic nephropathy, aggressive disease management in overt nephropathy may still delay progression to ESRD.

References

1. Bakris GL, Williams M, Dworkin L et al. Preserving renal function in adults with hypertension and diabetes: a consensus approach. National Kidney Foundation Hypertension and Diabetes Executive Committees Working Group. *Am J Kidney Dis* 2000; **36**: 646–61.

2. O'Connor PJ, Spann SJ, Woolf SH. Care of adults with type 2 diabetes mellitus: a review of the evidence. *J Fam Pract* 1998; **47** (Suppl): S13 S22.

3. Hoy W. Screening for renal disease and other chronic diseases in Aboriginal adults, and preliminary experience of a medical intervention program. *Nephrology* 1998; **4**: S90–S95.

4. Scheid DC, McCarthy LH, Lawler FH, Hamm RM, Reilly KE. Screening for microalbuminuria to prevent nephropathy in patients with diabetes: a systematic review of the evidence. *J Fam Pract* 2000; **50**: 661–8.

5. Airaksinen KEJ. Silent coronary artery disease in diabetes – a feature of autonomic neuropathy or accelerated atherosclerosis. *Diabetologia* 2001; **44**: 259–66.

6. Airaksinen KE. Early diagnosis of silent coronary artery disease in diabetic subjects are intense efforts worthwhile? *Swiss Med Wkly* 2001; **131**: 425–6.

7. Shah BV, Levey AS. Spontaneous changes in the rate of decline in reciprocal serum creatinine: errors in predicting the progression of renal disease from extrapolation of the slope. *J Am Soc Nephrol* 1992; **2**: 1186–91.

8. Ruggeneti P. Chronic proteinuric nephropathies: outcomes and response to treatment in a prospective cohort of 352 patients with different patterns of renal injury. *Am J Kidney Dis* 2000; **35**: 1155–65.

9. Peterson JC, Adler S, Burkart JM et al. Blood pressure control, proteinuria, and the progression of renal disease. The Modification of Diet in Renal Disease Study. *Ann Intern Med* 1995; **123**: 754–62.

10. Mogensen CE, Hansen KW, Pederson MM, Christensen CK. Renal factors influencing blood pressure threshold and choice of treatment for hypertension in IDDM. *Diabetes Care* 1991; **14** (Suppl 4): 13 26.

11. United Kingdom Prospective Diabetes Study (UKPDS) Group. Tight blood pressure control and risk of macrovascular and microvascular complications in type 2 diabetes: UKPDS 38. *BMJ* 1998; **317**: 703 13.

12. Giugliano D, Acampora R, Marfella R et al. Metabolic and cardiovascular effects of carvedilol and atenolol in non-insulin-dependent diabetes mellitus and hypertension. A randomized, controlled trial. *Ann Intern Med* 1999; **26**: 955 9.

13. The sixth report of the Joint National Committee on Prevention, Detection, Evaluation, and Treatment of High Blood Pressure. *Arch Intern Med* 1997; **157**: 2413–46.

14. 1999 Guidelines for the management of hypertension; memorandum to the World Health Organization/International society of hypertension meeting. Guidelines subcommittee. *J Hypertens* 1999; **17**: 151 83.

15. Lewis EJ, Hunsicker LG, Clarke WR et al. Renoprotective effect of the angiotensin-receptor antagonist irbesartan in patients with nephropathy due to type 2 diabetes. *N Engl J Med* 2001; **345**: 851 -60.

16. Brenner BM, Cooper ME, de Zeeuw D et al. Effects of losartan on renal and cardiovascular outcomes in patients with type 2 diabetes and nephropathy. *N Engl J Med* 2001; **345**: 861 9.

17. Ravid M, Lang R, Rachmani R, Lishner M. Long-term renoprotective effect of angiotensin-converting enzyme inhibition in non-insulin-dependent diabetes mellitus. A 7-year follow-up study. *Arch Intern Med* 1996; **156**: 286–9.

18. Randomised placebo-controlled trial of effect of ramipril on decline in glomerular filtration rate and risk of terminal failure in proteinuria, non-diabetic nephropathy. The GISEN group (Gruppo Italiano di Studi Epidemiologici in Nefrologia). *Lancet* 1997; **349**: 1857 -63.

19. Lebovitz HE, Wiegmann TB, Cnann A et al. Renal protective effects of enalapril in hypertensive NIDDM: role of baseline albuminuria. *Kidney Int* 1994; **45**(Suppl.): 150–5.

20. Nielsen S, Schmitz A, Moller N et al. Renal function and insulin sensitivity during simvastatin treatment in type 2 (non-insulin-dependent) diabetic patients with microalbuminuria. *Diabetologia* 1993; **36**: 1079–86.

21. Parving HH, Rossing P. The use of anti-hypertensive agents in prevention and treatment of diabetic nephropathy. *Curr Opin Nephrol Hypertens* 1994; **3**: 292–300.

22. Ruilope LM, Salvetti A, Jamerson K et al. Renal function and intensive lowering of blood pressure in hypertensive participants of the hypertension optimal treatment (HOT) study. *J Am Soc Nephrol* 2001; **12**: 218 -25.

23. Hansson L, Lindholm LH, Niskanen L et al. Effect of angiotensin-converting-enzyme inhibition compared with conventional therapy on cardiovascular morbidity and mortality in hypertension: the Captopril Prevention Project (CAPPP) randomised trial. *Lancet* 1999; **353**: 611–16.

24. Ferder L, Daccordi H, Martello M, Panzlis M, Inserra F. Angiotensin converting enzyme inhibitors versus calcium antagonists in the treatment of diabetic hypertensive patients. *Hypertension* 1992; **19** (Suppl 2): 237–42.

25. Weidmann P, Schneider M, Bohlen L. Effects of different antihypertensive drugs on human diabetic nephropathy: an updated META analysis. *Nephrol Dial Transpl* 1995; **10** (S9): 39–45.

26. Jerums G, Cooper ME, Gilbert RE, Atkins RC. Renal protection by angiotensin II receptor antagonists in patients with type 2 diabetes. *Med J Aust* 2001; **175**: 397–9.

27. Bakris GL, Mangrum A, Copley JB, Vicknair N, Sadler R. Effect of calcium channel or beta-blockade on the progression of diabetic nephropathy in African Americans. *Hypertension* 1997; **29**: 244–50.

28. Bakris GL, Weir MR, DeQuattro V, McMahon FG. Effects of an ACE inhibitor/calcium antagonist combination on proteinuria in diabetic nephropathy. *Kidney Int* 1998; **54**: 1283–9.

29. National Heart, Lung and Blood Institute/National Institute of Diabetes and Digestive and Kidney Diseases. *Clinical Guidelines on the Identification, Evaluation, and Treatment of Overweight and Obesity in Adults.* National Heart, Lung and Blood Institute, 1998.

30. Praga M, Hernandez E, Herero JC et al. Influence of obesity on the appearance of proteinuria and renal insufficiency after unilateral nephrectomy. *Kidney Int* 2000; **58**: 2111–18.

31. Praga M, Hernandez E, Andres A et al. Effects of body-weight loss and captopril treatment on proteinuria associated with obesity. *Nephron* 1995; **70**: 35–41.

32. Fleischmann E, Teal N, Dudley J et al. Influence of excess weight on mortality and hospital stay in 1346 haemodialysis patients. *Kidney Int* 1999; **55**: 1580–1.

151

33. Bjrck S. Clinical trials in overt diabetic nephropathy. In: Mogensen CE, ed. *The Kidney and Hypertension in Diabetes*, 3rd edn. The Netherlands: Kluwer Academic Publishers, 1997.

34. Parving HH. Renoprotection in diabetes: genetic and non-genetic risk factors and treatment. *Diabetologia* 1998; **41**: 745–59.

35. Kanoun F, Ben Amor Z, Zouari B, Ben Khalifa F. Insulin therapy may increase blood pressure levels in type 2 diabetes mellitus. *Diabetes Metab* 2001; **27**: 695–700.

36. Reardon LC, Macpherson DS. Hyperkalemia in outpatients using angiotensin-converting enzyme inhibitors: how much should we worry? *Arch Intern Med* 1998; **158**: 26–32.

37. Schepkens H, Vanholder R, Billiouw JM, Lameire N. Life-threatening hyperkalemia during combined therapy with angiotensin-converting enzyme inhibitors and spironolactone: an analysis of 25 cases. *Am J Med* 2000; **110**: 438–41.

38. ADRAC, Thomas MC, Mathew TH, Boyd I. Diuretics, ACE inhibitors and NSAIDs – the triple whammy. *Med J Aust* 2000; **172**: 184–5.

39. Parfrey PS, Griffiths SM, Barrett BJ. Contrast material-induced renal failure in patients with diabetes mellitus, renal insufficiency, or both. A prospective controlled study. *N Engl J Med* 1989; **320**: 143.

40. Rudnick MR, Goldfarb S, Wexler L et al. Nephrotoxicity of ionic and nonionic contrast media in 1196 patients: a randomized trial. The Iohexol Cooperative Study. *Kidney Int* 1995; **47**: 254–61.

41. Manske CL, Sprafka JM, Strong JH, Wang Y. Contrast nephropathy in azotemic diabetic patients undergoing coronary angiography. *Am J Med* 1990; **89**: 615.

42. Solomon R, Werner C, Mann D, D'Elia J, Silva P. Effects of saline, mannitol, and furosemide to prevent acute decreases in renal function induced by radiocontrast agents. *N Engl J Med* 1994; **331**: 1416.

43. Stevens MA, McCullough PA, Tobin KJ. A prospective randomized trial of prevention measures in patients at high risk for contrast nephropathy: results of the P.R.I.N.C.E. Study. Prevention of Radiocontrast Induced Nephropathy Clinical Evaluation. *J Am Coll Cardiol* 1999; **33**: 403–11.

44. Weisberg LS, Kurnik BR. Risk of radiocontrast nephropathy in patients with and without diabetes mellitus. *Kidney Int* 1994; **45**: 259–65.

45. Cigarroa RG, Lange RA, Williams RH, Hillia LD. Dosing of contrast material to prevent contrast nephropathy in patients with renal disease. *Am J Med* 1989; **86**: 649.

46. Tepel M, van der Giet M, Schwarzfeld C, Laufer U, Liermann D, Zidek W. Prevention of radiographic-contrast-agent-induced reductions in renal function by acetylcysteine. *N Engl J Med* 2000; **343**: 180–4.

47. Game FL, Bartlett WA, Bayly GR, Jones AF. Comparative accuracy of cardiovascular risk prediction methods in patients with diabetes mellitus. *Diabetes Obes Metab* 2001; **3**: 279–86.

CASE 33: DIABETES AND MICROALBUMINURIA: A MULTI-SYSTEM DISEASE

Michael Krimholtz, Stephen Thomas and Giancarlo Viberti

History

A Caucasian woman was diagnosed with type 2 diabetes and hypertension in 1973 at the age of 44 following a road traffic accident. The woman was obese with a BMI > 31 and predominantly central fat distribution. There were no complications at presentation. Treatment consisted of diet, oral hypoglycaemics and chlorthalidone for hypertension. Ten years after diagnosis, peripheral neuropathy and proliferative diabetic retinopathy were diagnosed, the latter requiring photocoagulation. In 1988, aged 59 and 15 years after diagnosis, insulin therapy was commenced for deteriorating glycaemic control. She was referred to the Diabetes Centre in 1991. By then antihypertensive therapy had been discontinued and the insulin regimen consisted of twice daily Human Mixtard (30/70); HbA1c was 6.2%. Her sitting blood pressure (BP) was 200/94 mmHg and standing BP was 170/76 mmHg. Absent pedal pulses were documented. Her total cholesterol was 7.7 mmol/L (LDL 6.7 mmol/L, HDL 1.0 mmol/L, HDL/total cholesterol ratio 0.13) and triglyceride 2.27 mmol/L. Microalbuminuria was documented with an albumin excretion rate (AER) of 162 µg/min. She was started on a low-fat diet and her insulin dose was reduced because of mid-morning hypoglycaemic attacks. An angiotensin-converting enzyme inhibitor (ACEI) was commenced. Over the next year glycaemic control remained stable, HbA1c 7.1%, and BP had fallen to 178/88. A reduced glomerular filtration rate (GFR) was documented (^{51}Cr EDTA clearance 73 ml/min/1.73 m^2), although serum creatinine was normal at 89 µmol/L. A left pars plana was performed with further photocoagulation and bilateral cataract extractions, and chronic open angle glaucoma had been diagnosed. Treatment consisted of ACEI and the newly licensed HMG CoA reductase inhibitor.

Over the next 2 years her BMI increased to 32 and glycaemic control deteriorated with HbA1c between 9% and 11%. Total cholesterol levels averaged 5.8 mmol/L with triglyceride levels 1.3 mmol/L. Sitting BP levels averaged 160/76 mmHg despite antihypertensive treatment with ACEIs and the addition of a thiazide diuretic. The AER rose to around 600 µg/min and conventional protein dipstick tests became positive. The ^{51}Cr EDTA GFR feel to 64 ml/min/m^2 although the serum creatinine remained within the normal range at 86 µmol/L. Renal ultrasound showed a right kidney of 11.5 cm and a slightly smaller left kidney of 10 cm in size. Symptoms of carpal tunnel syndrome had developed and surgical decompression was performed.

In 1994, 21 years after diagnosis, she developed angina at the age of 67, and a β-blocker and aspirin were added to the therapy. A standard 12-lead electrocardiograph was consistent with ischemia. On coronary angiography there was diffuse disease of both the left anterior descending and right coronary arteries with multiple stenoses and significant left ventricular hypertrophy was also present.

The glycaemic control remained suboptimal with HbA1c ~ 9% despite insulin and metformin therapy. Systolic BP remained elevated at 152/70 mmHg despite ACEI, diuretic, β-blocker and calcium antagonist (CCB) therapy.

By 2001, 28 years after diagnosis, at the age of 72, the patient developed biventricular failure and the serum creatinine had risen to 136 µmol/L, after which the metformin was discontinued.

Her peripheral vascular disease worsened and she developed a neuroischaemic foot ulcer that required intravenous antibiotic treatment. Doppler angiology confirmed extensive proximal and distal peripheral vascular disease. Currently her total cholesterol is 3.9 µmol/L, her HbA1c is in the range 9–10%, BMI 40.7, GFR 37 ml/min/m^2, AER 116 mg/day. Serum potassium ranges between 5.1 and 5.7 mmol/L. Her BP is around 138/50. Her treatment consists of a basal bolus insulin regimen, lisinopril 10 mg, bisoprolol 5 mg, felodipine 10 mg, bumetanide 2 mg, bendrofluazide 2.5 mg, simvastatin 40 mg OD, nicorandil and GTN spray.

In summary this Caucasian woman presented as a chance diagnosis of type 2 diabetes and hypertension at the age of 44. Over the next 15 years there were progressive microvascular complications including the development of microalbuminuria, and latterly peripheral neuropathy, renal failure and proliferative diabetic retinopathy. These have been followed by progressive macrovascular complications with coronary artery disease, biventricular failure and peripheral vascular disease.

Commentary

The relationship between microalbuminuria and hypertension in type 2 diabetes was first described in the late 1960s.[1] Since then several authors have described the strong association between microalbuminuria and cardiovascular (CV) risk factors and CV morbidity.[2]

The absolute risk of CV death for people with type 2 diabetes is two to four times higher and progressively greater with each additional risk factor than in non-diabetic patients.[3] In fact, the risk of a first myocardial infarction in an individual with diabetes is as great as that of a non-diabetic individual with a previous myocardial infarction.[4] Furthermore, the increase in risk is particularly marked in females. The patient with type 2 diabetes who develops microalbuminuria has a further 2–3-fold increase in the risk of CV event compared with the patient who remains normoalbuminuric.[5] Thus microalbuminuria in this patient population is not only a marker of kidney disease, and a risk factor for progressive renal failure, but also a strong predictor of CV morbidity and mortality.

The Hypertension Optimal Treatment (HOT) study has suggested that the lowest risk of major cardiovascular events in subjects with hypertension occurred at BP values of approximately 139/80 mmHg.[6] Recent JNC VI recommendations suggest an aim in diabetes for a BP of 130/85.[7] The most common form of hypertension in type 2 diabetes, as illustrated by this case, is a rise in systolic pressure with a widening of pulse pressure. There is growing evidence that systolic hypertension and large pulse pressure excursions may be particularly damaging to the kidney. Optimal BP treatment can be problematic and, as seen in the case, may require different antihypertensive drugs. In this patient four different antihypertensives were used and yet by modern recommendations systolic BP never returned to within target values. This is consistent with the data from the hypertension in diabetes arm of the UKPDS where an average of three different antihypertensive drugs were required to achieve a mean time-averaged BP over 9 years of 144/82.[8]

The optimal use and dosage of antihypertensive drugs in diabetes and particularly in diabetic kidney disease (DKD) is still the subject of debate. This patient's treatment comprised primarily an ACE inhibitor with upward titration of the dose followed by the addition of a diuretic. This combination produced a BP fall of 40 mmHg in systolic and 18 mmHg in diastolic BP. There is evidence, over and above the beneficial effect of BP lowering, for a specific renal and cardioprotective benefit of ACE inhibitors in this type of patient. Diuretics, as well as low salt intake, potentiate the effect of ACE inhibitors and are useful in their own right, as hypertension in diabetes (and particularly in DKD) is often salt-sensitive. The addition of a β-blocker and a CCB further lowered BP by approximately 12 and 5 mmHg for systolic and diastolic BP, respectively. CCBs are often effective in controlling systolic hypertension but there are data that indicate that dihydropyridine CCBs, such as the one prescribed to this patient, may be less cardioprotective and renoprotective when used as primary monotherapy. There is no evidence, however, that when used in combination with ACE inhibitors they hinder the ACE inhibitors' beneficial effect.

Despite multiple antihypertensive drug therapy this patient developed progressive renal failure and cardiovascular disease. Some authors argue,[9] that the ACE inhibitor should be increased to the maximum tolerated dose for optimal effect. This manoeuvre is often hampered (as in this case) by the tendency to develop high serum potassium levels secondary to abnormalities in renal tubular potassium handling. For this reason the combination of an ACE inhibitor and an AII receptor antagonist (AIIA), which has been proposed recently as a strategy for remission of renal disease, was not considered. Two recent controlled trials in patients with type 2 diabetes with various degrees of DKD have demonstrated that therapy with an angiotensin II receptor antagonist has renoprotective effects largely independent of BP lowering. However, these trials showed no protection against coronary artery disease and cerebrovascular disease, although there was a reduction in hospital admissions for chronic heart failure.[10,11] It remains arguable whether AIIA would have been more efficacious than ACEI.

The presence of asymmetric kidney sizes suggests reno-vascular disease, but no acute deterioration of renal function was seen on initiation and increase of ACE inhibition, as may have been expected if any clinically relevant artery stenosis was present. In the future, investigation with renal angiography or MR angiography may be necessary. Higher rates of proteinuria are associated with, and probably a determinant of, rates of renal disease progression and higher CV morbidity/mortality. Therapy in these patients should be directed to achieve maximal anti-proteinuric effect. Albuminuria < 0.3 mg/day has been suggested to indicate regression of proteinuric chronic nephropathies.[9] Unfortunately, in this case this was not associated with stabilization of renal function, which continued to deteriorate.

Lipid-lowering treatment is also a key intervention in these patients for reduction of CV mortality,[12,13] but there are no controlled data on the effect of this therapy on renal disease progression in diabetes. The guidelines for ideal lipid levels in diabetes have tightened recently with a recommendation in patients like this for total cholesterol < 5.0 mmol/L (LDL < 3.0 mmol/L, HDL > 1.4 mmol/L) triglyceride <1.5 mmol/L.[14]

In summary, aggressive multi-drug therapy may be necessary, targeted at different CV risk factors, with new more recent targets of treatment. This highlights the severity of type 2 diabetes as a vascular disease. Although in the light of recent recommendations, aspects of this patient's treatment may have been different (which may have delayed progression), this case also illustrates the need for a continued search for new treatment modalities if protection of target organ damage is to be achieved at an individual level.

References

1. Keen H, Chlouverakis C, Fuller J, Jarrett RJ. The concomitants of raised blood sugar: studies in newly-detected hyperglycaemics. II. Urinary albumin excretion, blood pressure and their relation to blood sugar levels. *Guys Hospital Reports* 1969; 118: 247–54.

2. Mattock MB, Barnes DJ, Viberti G et al. Microalbuminuria and coronary heart disease in NIDDM: an incidence study. *Diabetes* 1998; **47**: 1786–92.

3. Stamler J, Vaccaro O, Neaton JD, Wentworth D. Diabetes, other risk factors, and 12-yr cardiovascular mortality for men screened in the Multiple Risk Factor Intervention Trial. *Diabetes Care* 1993; **16**: 434–44.

4. Haffner SM, Lehto S, Ronnemaa T, Pyorala K, Laakso M. Mortality from coronary heart disease in subjects with type 2 diabetes and in nondiabetic subjects with and without prior myocardial infarction. *N Engl J Med* 1998; **339**: 229–34.

5. Macleod JM, Lutale J, Marshall SM. Albumin excretion and vascular deaths in NIDDM. *Diabetologia* 1995; **38**: 610–6.

6. Hansson L, Zanchetti A, Carruthers SG et al. Effects of intensive blood-pressure lowering and low-dose aspirin in patients with hypertension: principal results of the Hypertension Optimal Treatment (HOT) randomised trial. *Lancet* 2001; **351**: 1755–62.

7. Elliott WJ, Weir DR, Black HR. Cost-effectiveness of the lower treatment goal (of JNC VI) for diabetic hypertensive patients. Joint National Committee on Prevention, Detection, Evaluation, and Treatment of High Blood Pressure. *Arch Intern Med* 2000; **160**: 1277–83.

8. UKPDS Prospective Diabetes Study (UKPDS) Group. Tight blood pressure control and risk of macrovascular and microvascular complications in type 2 diabetes: UKPDS 38. UK Prospective Diabetes Study Group. *BMJ* 1998; **317**: 703–13.

9. Ruggenenti P, Schieppati A, Remuzzi G. Progression, remission, regression of chronic renal diseases. *Lancet* 2001; **357**: 1601–8.

10. Elkeles RS, Diamond JR, Poulter C et al. Cardiovascular outcomes in type 2 diabetes. A double-blind placebo-controlled study of bezafibrate: the St Mary's, Ealing, Northwick Park Diabetes Cardiovascular Disease Prevention (SENDCAP) Study. *Diabetes Care* 1998; **21**: 641–8.

11. Davis TM, Parsons RW, Broadhurst RJ, Hobbs MS, Jamrozik K. Arrhythmias and mortality after myocardial infarction in diabetic patients. Relationship to diabetes treatment. *Diabetes Care* 1998; **21**: 637–40.

12. Haffner SM. The Scandinavian Simvastatin Survival Study (4S) subgroup analysis of diabetic subjects: implications for the prevention of coronary heart disease. *Diabetes Care* 1997; **20**: 469–71.

13. Lewis SJ, Sacks FM, Mitchell JS et al. Effect of proavastatin on cardiovascular events in women after myocardial infarction: the cholesterol and recurrent events (CARE) trial. *J Am Coll Cardiol* 1998; **32**: 140–6.

14. Wood D, Durrington PN, Poulter NR et al. Joint British recommendations on prevention of coronary heart disease in clinical practice. *Heart* 1998; **80**(Suppl. 2): S1–S29.

CASE 34: DIABETES AND DYSBETALIPOPROTEINAEMIA

James Best, Myra Yeo and Andrew MacIsaac

History

AD was a 31-year-old Caucasian male, when in 1986 he was referred to a renal physician because of proteinuria, noted during a medical examination for insurance purposes. There was no significant personal or family history of kidney disease. He was 92 kg and 175 cm tall, with body mass index (BMI) 30.0 kg/m². Laboratory investigations reported creatinine 0.09 mmol/L, urea 7.9 mmol/L, urinary protein 4.54 g/day, fasting plasma glucose 6.0 mmol/L, total cholesterol 8.8 mmol/L, triglyceride 10.4 mmol/L, LDL-cholesterol 1.9 mmol/L and HDL-cholesterol 0.5 mmol/L. Both apoE phenotype and genotype were confirmed as E2/E2, and a renal biopsy showed widespread fat infiltration of glomerular cells. On further clinical examination, there were no xanthomas, xanthelasma or arcus senilis. He was treated with a diet low in saturated fat, clofibrate and later simvastatin.

Five years later, in 1991, he re-presented with episodic epigastric pain. On examination, he now weighed 101 kg (BMI 33.0 kg/m²), his blood pressure was 140/90 mmHg and hepatosplenomegaly was noted. His total cholesterol was 10.5 mmol/L with triglyceride 20.2 mmol/L and HDL-cholesterol 0.6 mmol/L. Amylase was elevated at 173 IU/L (normal 35–140) and a CT scan of his abdomen showed an enlarged liver, with fat infiltration, an enlarged spleen of 18 cm length and inflammatory changes consistent with pancreatitis involving the pancreatic tail. Random plasma glucose levels were 12.2 mmol/L and 16.2 mmol/L. He was commenced on gemfibrozil, and the symptoms resolved after 3 days. Advice was given on a diet low in saturated fat and with reduced energy. Three months following the admission, fasting plasma glucose level was noted to be 9.3 mmol/L, with HbA1c 5.8%, total cholesterol 6.8 mmol/L, triglyceride 8.0 mmol/L and HDL-cholesterol 0.9 mmol/L. The sulphonylurea glipizide was commenced 6 months later because of persistent hyperglycaemia.

In 1997, at the age of 42 years, AD continued to have poorly controlled combined hyperlipidaemia and diabetes. Despite treatment with glibenclamide, metformin and gemfibrozil, his HBA1c was 11.8%, total cholesterol 9.2 mmol/L and triglyceride 8.9 mmol/L. He was commenced on night-time NPH insulin when his body weight was 101 kg. He had commenced treatment with low-dose aspirin and his blood pressure was elevated at 155/90 mmHg. He worked as a cleaner and frequently mentioned that he was under considerable stress because of staff restructuring and external contracting.

A year after the initiation of insulin, his weight had increased to 103 kg (BMI 33.6 kg/m^2). An ophthalmology review reported no evidence of retinopathy, but urinary protein excretion was 5.89 g/day, with plasma creatinine level 0.08 mmol/L. He also developed intermittent chest pain with normal resting ECG, but a positive exercise stress test. The coronary angiogram showed diffuse disease and an 80% stenosis in the right coronary artery, which was stented (Figure 1a). Treatment with atorvastatin and diltiazem was subsequently initiated, while his insulin requirement rose from 20 to 72 units of night-time NPH insulin over the 12-month period.

In early 1999, he weighed 109 kg (BMI 35.6 kg/m^2) and blood pressure was 150/95 mmHg. HbA1c was 9.5%, total cholesterol 4.5 mmol/L, triglyceride 6.4 mmol/L, HDL 0.76 mmol/L. Urinary protein excretion was 2.88 g/day. Medications consisted of NPH insulin, glibenclamide, metformin, ramipril, atorvastatin, gemfibrozil, diltiazem and aspirin. Glibenclamide was reduced in an attempt to reduce his increasing weight, and irbesartan was introduced instead of ramipril because of the development of a cough. He complained of sexual dysfunction but a trial of sildenafil produced little improvement. Testosterone, prolactin, FSH and LH levels were normal, as were thyroid function tests. He expressed frustration about his multiple medical problems and the multiple medications required.

In early 2001 AD weighed 110 kg (BMI 35.9 kg/m^2) and his blood pressure was 145/85 mmHg. Waist circumference was 122 cm and waist-to-hip ratio was 1.07. He had mild non-proliferative retinopathy in both eyes. HbA1c was 9.9%, cholesterol 4.8 mmol/L, triglyceride 5.5 mmol/L and HDL-cholesterol 0.73 mmol/L. Urinary albumin excretion was 3.9 g/day, creatinine clearance rate was 2.49 ml/s and plasma creatinine 0.09 mmol/L. He was taking atenolol, amlodipine and irbesartan plus hydrochlorothiazide for his hypertension; gemfibrozil and atorvastatin for his combined hyperlipidaemia; insulin, metformin and glibenclamide for his diabetes and aspirin. He was commenced on pioglitazone 15 mg daily and then 30 mg daily to achieve better glycaemic control. His night-time NPH insulin was reduced from 80 to 60 units. HbA1c fell to 9.2% and lipid profile showed cholesterol 6.0 mmol/L, triglyceride 5.9 mmol/L and HDL-cholesterol 0.97 mmol/L. His weight increased to 115 kg (BMI 37.5 kg/m^2) and he was concerned that his face appeared 'puffy'. He did not want to see a dietitian for assessment or advice.

Because of weight gain and development of moderate ankle oedema, pioglitazone was stopped. HbA1c rose to 11.3%, triglyceride level to 10.3 mmol/L, weight to 116 kg and blood pressure to 160/90. He developed exertional chest tightness and was admitted to hospital for coronary angiogram and review of his diabetes. The angiogram showed extensive coronary artery stenoses, not readily amenable to bypass graft surgery (Figure 1b). Left

160

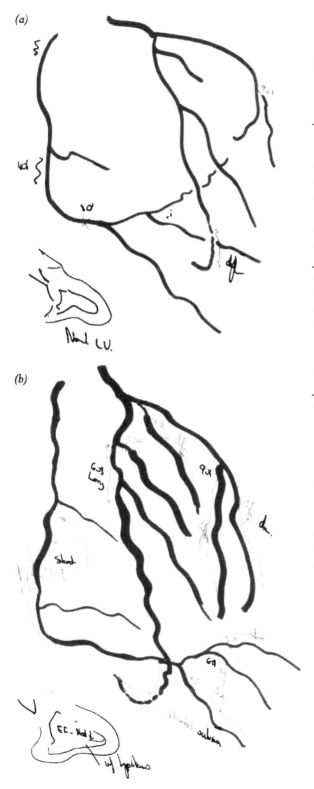

Figure 1 Coronary angiogram results for this patient with diabetes and dysbetalipoproteinaemia. (Ventriculogram showed normal left ventricular function on both occasions.) (a) April 1998. Left main trunk normal. Left anterior descending (LAD) system is disease-free in its proximal and mid regions, but has diffuse disease at the cardiac apex. The circumflex artery is a small vessel, with a small first obtuse marginal, which has a 90% stenosis at its ostium. The right coronary artery (RCA) is a huge dominant vessel with diffuse disease proximally, a 40% stenosis in the mid-anterior atrio-ventricular groove, a further 80% stenosis just proximal to the crux and minor distal disease. The 80% RCA stenosis was stented. (b) LAD has a mid-vessel 70–80% stenosis with distal diffuse disease. The RCA has proximal to mid-vessel tight stenosis. There is tight stenosis at the proximal diagonal artery ostium and a tight stenosis of the left ventricular branch.

161

ventricular function was normal. Assessment by a dietitian revealed that he had a high intake of saturated fat. Insulin therapy was changed to twice daily 50% regular/50% NPH insulin and over the next 2 months his weight fell to 113 kg, HbA1c to 9.9% and triglyceride level to 5.5 mmol/L. Blood pressure was 138/90.

Commentary

AD has the classical features of the insulin resistance syndrome.[1,2] He is obese, with a central distribution of body fat, has hypertension, elevated triglyceride and low HDL-cholesterol levels and diabetes. At 43 years of age, he developed symptomatic coronary heart disease that has progressed significantly over the following 4 years.

The unusual aspect of his diabetes is the severe nature of the associated dyslipidaemia. The prevalence of homozygosity for apolipoprotein E2 (E2/E2 genotype) is about 1% in Western populations[3] and in most studies of type 2 diabetes there is no increase in frequency of E2. The common allele is apolipoprotein E3 and so the usual genotype is E3/E3. Apolipoprotein E2 has lower affinity for the hepatic receptors that remove intermediate density lipoprotein particles (intermediate in size and composition between very low density and low density lipoprotein particles and so rich in both triglyceride and cholesterol) from the circulation. However, only about 2% of individuals with apolipoprotein E2/E2 genotype develop the clinical phenotype of type III hyperlipoproteinaemia or dysbetalipoproteinaemia.[4] Expression of the clinical phenotype in genetically predisposed individuals requires the presence of an additional inherited or acquired lipid disorder, such as familial combined hyperlipidaemia[5] or hypothyroidism. Given the severity of the dyslipidaemia, it is possible that he has the additional genetically determined lipid disorder of familial combined hyperlipidaemia,[5] but there is no specific laboratory test for this condition. Type 2 diabetes may be an aggravating factor, as it is associated with elevated triglycerides and low HDL-cholesterol.[6] In this case the lipid abnormalities preceded the onset of hyperglycaemia, but the dyslipidaemia of type 2 diabetes does often precede the onset of diabetes.[7]

Dysbetalipoproteinaemia is associated with greatly increased risk for coronary heart disease, as has occurred at an early age in this patient. It generally responds well to treatment with fibric acid derivatives[8] and HMG CoA reductase inhibitors can also be effective,[9] but in this case triglyceride and HDL-cholesterol levels remained significantly abnormal despite treatment with both gemfibrozil and atorvastatin. Some improvement did result from the addition of pioglitazone therapy, a PPARγ agonist that has been shown to enhance insulin sensitivity and improve diabetic dyslipidaemia.[10] Experimental evidence indicates several other potentially anti-atherogenic actions of PPARγ agonists,[11] but there are no clinical outcome studies. Unfortunately, these agents can also lead to weight gain from peripheral fat deposition and to peripheral oedema, as occurred in this patient. Despite knowing that there was a high risk for development of atherosclerotic vascular disease in this patient, preventive measures have not been able to stop the development of severe coronary heart disease. However, it is possible that treatment has prevented myocardial infarction or coronary mortality.

The marked dyslipidaemia caused several other complications in this patient, including a very unusual form of renal disease, the reason for his initial presentation.[12] Significant proteinuria and dyslipidaemia persist 15 years later but creatinine clearance remains normal and there is no indication for a further renal biopsy. Other complications that resulted from the dyslipidaemia were pancreatitis and hepatosplenomegaly, which can result from fat infiltration in dysbetalipoproteinaemia. Both conditions resolved with lipid-modifying therapy.

The main management challenge in treating this patient has been his inability to maintain dietary restrictions and the need for polypharmacy. He works as a cleaner, starting work at 3:00 am and has been constantly concerned over the past few years that he will lose his job, as have many of his colleagues, through contracting out of most of the cleaning services. The patient has frequently felt discouraged because of his continuing weight gain and the need for so much medication. He was particularly discouraged by the diagnosis of ischaemic heart disease. On several occasions, he has expressed the view that he 'might as well stop everything'. Initiation of insulin and later pioglitazone has been associated with further weight gain. He has generally been reluctant to see dietitians, but did so during his recent hospital admission and there has been some short-term weight reduction. Treatment with a very low calorie diet either in hospital or out of hospital has been declined because of concern about missing work or not having enough energy to work, and also because of the expense. Besides, there is no evidence that this approach will be effective long term.

What did I learn from this case?

What has been learned from this patient is to negotiate carefully each change in medication and to tackle one issue at a time, such as glycaemic control, dyslipidaemia or hypertension. His obesity is clearly a key issue, but focusing too much on his weight causes him to become agitated. It has been important to remain encouraging in order to maintain morale, although informing the patient of health risk is justified.[13] Working with his general practitioner, who has known him since childhood and shares the same ethnic background, has been very helpful to maintain contact with the patient and to convince him to continue with the large number of medications. This case epitomises the frustration for patient and physician of requiring multiple medications to treat multiple, but linked conditions and emphasises the refractory nature of obesity.

References

1. Kaplan NM. The deadly quartet: upper body obesity, glucose intolerance, hypertriglyceridemia, and hypertension. *Arch Intern Med* 1989; **149**: 1514–20.

2. DeFronzo RA, Ferrannini E. Insulin resistance. A multifaceted syndrome responsible for NIDDM, obesity, hypertension, dyslipidemia, and atherosclerotic cardiovascular disease. *Diabetes Care* 1991; **14**: 173–94.

3. Assmann G, Schmitz G, Menzel HJ, Schulte H. Apolipoprotein E polymorphism and hyperlipidemia. *Clin Chem* 1984; **30**: 641–3.

4. Mahley RW, Rall SC Jr. Type III hyperlipoproteinemia (dysbetalipoproteinemia): the role of apolipoprotein E in normal and abnormal lipoprotein metabolism. In: Scriver CR, Beaudet AL, Sly WS, Valle D, eds. *The Metabolic and Molecular Bases of Inherited Disease.* New York: McGraw Hill, 1995: 1953–80.

5. Kane JP, Havel RJ. Disorders of the biogenesis and secretion of lipoproteins containing the B apolipoproteins. In: Scriver CR, Beaudet AL, Sly WS, Valle D, eds. *The Metabolic and Molecular Bases of Inherited Disease.* New York: McGraw Hill, 1995: 1853–85.

6. UK Prospective Diabetes Study (UKPDS). XI: Biochemical risk factors in type 2 diabetic patients at diagnosis compared with age-matched normal subjects. *Diabetic Med* 1994; **11**: 534–44.

7. Haffner SM, Stern MP, Hazuda HP, Mitchell BD, Patterson JK. Cardiovascular risk factors in confirmed prediabetic individuals. Does the clock for coronary heart disease start ticking before the onset of clinical diabetes? *JAMA* 1990; **263**: 2893 8.

8. Zhao SP, Smelt AH, Leuven JA, Vroom TF, van der Lasse A, van't Hooft FM. Changes of lipoprotein profile in familial dysbetalipoproteinemia with gemfibrozil. *Am J Med* 1994; **96**: 49 56.

9. Feussner G, Eichinger M, Ziegler R. The influence of simvastatin alone or in combination with gemfibrozil on plasma lipids and lipoproteins in patients with Type III hyperlipoproteinemia. *Clin Invest* 1992; **70**: 1027–35.

10. Aronoff S, Rosenblatt S, Braithwaite S, Egan JW, Mathisen AL, Schneider RL. The Pioglitazone 001 Study Group. Pioglitazone hydrochloride monotherapy improves glycemic control in the treatment of patients with type 2 diabetes: a 6 month randomized placebo-controlled dose-response study. *Diabetes Care* 2000; **23**: 1605 11.

11. Hsueh WA, Law RE. PPARgamma and atherosclerosis: effects on cell growth and movement. *Arterioscler Thromb Vasc Biol* 2001; **21**: 1891 5.

12. Balson KR, Niall JF, Best JD. Glomerular lipid deposition and proteinuria in a patient with familial dysbetalipoproteinaemia. *J Intern Med* 1996; **240**: 157–9.

13. Becker MH, Janz NK. Behavioural science perspectives on health hazard/health risk appraisal. *Health Serv Res* 1987; **22**: 537–51.

Case 35: Type 2 Diabetes Presenting with an Itchy Rash

Gerry Fegan and John E Tooke

History

A 50-year-old male presented to his general practitioner with a 2-week history of a pruritic papular rash affecting his elbows, knees and buttocks. He complained of lethargy but denied any polyuria, polydipsia or weight loss. He was treated with a 1-week trial of topical steroids with no improvement.

There was no past medical history or family history of note. The patient had a sedentary lifestyle and consumed a diet high in saturated fat. His alcohol intake was 16 units weekly and he did not smoke.

Examination and investigations

On examination the patient was centrally obese with a body mass index of 32 kg/m². Raised pruritic lesions were present over his extensor surfaces; they appeared yellow in colour (Figure 1). He was hypertensive with a blood

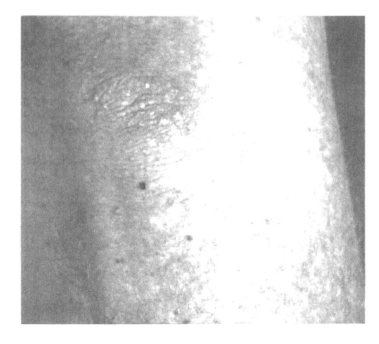

Figure 1
Eruptive
xanthomata.

pressure of 152/95 mmHg. His abdomen was soft and fundoscopy was normal.

Blood sampling revealed lipaemic serum (Figure 2) and laboratory investigations were as follows: plasma glucose 22 mmol/L, total cholesterol 56 mmol/L, triglycerides > 100 mmol/L, amylase normal and sodium 156 mmol/L (pseudohypernatraemia).

Figure 2 Lipaemic serum.

Diagnosis

1. Eruptive xanthomata
2. Acute hypertriglyceridaemia
3. Type 2 diabetes/insulin resistance
4. Obesity.

Treatment and outcome

The patient was reviewed at the Diabetes Centre on the same day that the biochemical investigations were carried out. Initially advice was given to avoid foods high in saturated fats and sugar, and he was treated with metformin and a fibric acid derivative. The hypertriglyceridaemia, hyperglycaemia and rash did not improve over the next 3 days and he developed ketonuria (++ urine) but no metabolic acidosis. Isophane insulin was then added with dramatic improvement of the rash, glucose and lipids. Initially 48 units twice daily were required but as the metabolic derangement improved the insulin therapy was discontinued safely 2 weeks later. Metformin and fibrate therapies were also successfully withdrawn over the next 3 months. He now continues on HMG CoA reductase inhibitor alone, with a HbA1c of 4.8% and normal cholesterol and triglycerides.

Commentary

This patient represents an unusual presentation of type 2 diabetes. His 'itchy rash', initially treated with topical steroids, was eruptive xanthomata – reflecting the underlying severe hypertriglyceridaemia. The presence of the large macromolecular lipoproteins, chylomicrons, resulted in lipaemic serum and although both lipaemia retinalis and pancreatitis are also recognized complications of chylomicronaemia, this patient did not demonstrate them.

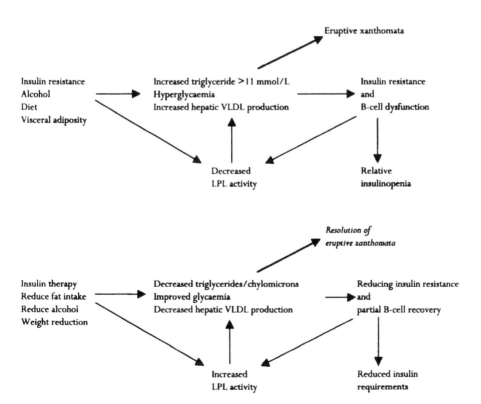

Figure 3 *Proposed cycles for the metabolic abnormalities before and after therapy.*

It is unlikely that a monogenic disorder accounts for the lipid abnormalities, given that normal lipids had been recorded by his general practitioner before presentation. Many mechanisms may have contributed to the severe dyslipidaemia observed in this patient, but it is likely that insulin resistance played a central role, and perhaps at the time of presentation a degree of insulinopenia (with the presence of moderate ketonuria). The activity of lipoprotein lipase (LPL), an endothelial enzyme which hydrolyses triglycerides, is impaired in type 2 diabetes and apolipoprotein C-III, an inhibitor of LPL, is elevated. This reduces the ability to clear exogenous triglyceride, and with increased circulating free fatty acids, hepatic production of VLDL (endogenous triglyceride) also increases. The LPL enzyme system becomes saturated and, with the dual defect of increased production and decreased clearance of triglyceride-rich lipoproteins, hypertriglyceridaemia and chylomicronaemia occur. A vicious circle of metabolic decompensation follows (Figure 3).

The interesting aspect of this case is how therapy influenced the metabolic improvement. The early introduction of insulin may, by activating LPL and interrupting the vicious circle, allow more rapid and effective correction of the acute hypertriglyceridaemia and the subsequent eruptive xanthomata.

What did I learn from this case?

Two learning points come from this case. First, when presented with an unusual itchy rash on the extensor surfaces consider eruptive xanthomata. This can be the first presentation of type 2 diabetes which reflects severe hypertriglyceridaemia. Second, the early use of insulin, at least in the short term, should be considered in these patients.

Further reading

Betteridge DJ. Diabetic dyslipidaemia. *Am J Med* 1994; **96** (Suppl 6A): 25S–31S.

Brunzell JD, Bierman MD. Chylomicronaemia syndrome. *Med Clin North Am* 1982; **66**: 455–68.

Case 36: Patient with Combined Hyperlipidaemia

Dirk Müller-Wieland and Wilhelm Krone

History

A 56-year-old patient was initially seen by his GP who referred him to the dermatology outpatient clinic because of his chief complaint, i.e. an unexplained rash with increasing intensity over recent weeks at his elbows and buttocks. Otherwise he felt healthy, there was no other concomitant disease known and he was not taking any regular medication. The social history revealed that he liked to play soccer at the weekend (in a so-called old men's team), which was associated with regular and increased alcohol consumption on these occasions. The family history showed that both parents are obese and suffer from type 2 diabetes, diagnosed when they were in their fifties.

Examination and investigations

The patient had tubero-eruptive xanthomas on both elbows and both buttocks as well as on his knees and was obese.

Laboratory investigations revealed elevated fasting triglycerides of 1200 mg/dL and total cholesterol 458 mg/dL. Ultracentrifugation was performed, revealing an HDL-cholesterol level of 35 mg/dL and LDL-cholesterol of 185 mg/dL. Fasting blood glucose was 95 mg/dL, but an oral glucose tolerance test showed a 2-h value of 265 mg/dL, HbA1c 6.8%.

Diagnosis

Tubero-eruptive xanthomas due to exacerbation of triglyceride levels as a result of combined hyperlipidaemia in association with type 2 diabetes.

Treatment and outcome

The patient received dietary recommendations. He was asked to reduce weight, first by about 5 kg. To reduce associated risk of pancreatitis the patient was initially treated with a fibrate and asked to avoid alcohol completely. After

4 weeks the skin rash was almost gone, he had already reduced his body weight by 3 kg and did not drink any alcohol. Triglyceride levels were reduced to 250 mg/dL, the LDL-cholesterol increased to 210 with an HDL-cholesterol of 38 mg/dL. After 6 months he had reduced weight by a total of 9 kg, the triglyceride levels were 180 mg/dL, LDL-cholesterol was 170 mg/dL, HDL-cholesterol 42. After 6 months of therapy, combination therapy with a statin was recommended in order to lower LDL-cholesterol levels below 100 mg/dL. Blood glucose levels were in the normal range and HbA1c was 6.2%.

Commentary

This is a typical case of a patient presenting with severe dyslipoproteinaemia as the first sign of a type 2 diabetes. Furthermore, it is typical in that triglyceride levels can be exacerbated – for example, by obesity and concomitant alcohol excess – to levels which lead to tubero-eruptive xanthomas, typically triglyceride levels are above 1000 mg/dl. Therefore, the first presenting complaint is a rash, which leads the patient to the dermatologist. This rash is usually reversible by triglyceride lowering. The key approach to the treatment of high triglyceride levels in patients with the so-called metabolic syndrome is the reduction of body weight, abstinence from alcohol and glucose control. Reduction of body weight by only about 5–10% has already had dramatic effects on increasing insulin sensitivity and thereby triglyceride lowering. As dyslipoproteinaemia is a very early and sensitive sign of the insulin resistance syndrome, the American Diabetes Association recommends screening this high risk population using an oral glucose tolerance test.

What are the essentials of lipid disorders in patients with insulin resistance and/or type 2 diabetes? About half of all patients with type 2 diabetes have a dyslipoproteinaemia. Typical alterations of plasma lipids are high triglyceride levels associated with low HDL-cholesterol levels (dyslipoproteinaemia) and possibly high LDL-cholesterol levels. Elevated LDL-cholesterol levels can be caused by reduced degradation via the LDL-receptor, which is regulated by insulin, as well as by modification of LDL-particles, e.g. glycolisation, increased oxidation and increased triglyceride content. These structural alterations of the LDL-particles, i.e. smaller and denser, are a key feature of insulin resistance and appear to increase the atherogenic potential of these particles. Therefore, patients with type 2 diabetes or metabolic syndrome appear to have a higher atherogenic risk at certain LDL-cholesterol levels compared with non-diabetics. As regards low HDL-cholesterol concentrations, it must be kept in mind that HDL metabolism is closely related to the metabolism of triglyceride-rich lipoproteins. Therefore it is a typical constellation, in that high triglyceride levels are associated with reduced HDL concentrations. Hypertriglyceridaemia on the basis of insulin resistance is commonly caused by an elevation of VLDL-particles. This can be due to an increased rate of synthesis and/or reduced rate of degradation.

Every patient with diabetes mellitus should know his plasma lipids. Therefore plasma levels of triglycerides, total cholesterol and HDL-cholesterol should be determined. According to the Friedewald formula LDL-cholesterol levels are the result of total cholesterol minus HDL-cholesterol minus triglyceride ÷ 5. The plasma triglycerides have to be divided by 5, because in the fasting state, high triglyceride levels are most likely due to elevated VLDL-particles, which usually carry 20% of cholesterol. Therefore, in a patient with high triglyceride levels, concomitant elevated total cholesterol levels are often not due to increased LDL-cholesterol, but to raised VLDL-cholesterol levels. It should be noted that HDL-cholesterol levels cannot be determined adequately, and therefore the Friedewald formula cannot be used, when triglyceride levels are higher than 400 mg/dl. In this case ultracentrifugation should be used to determine the lipoprotein concentrations correctly.

As there is epidemiological evidence that cardiovascular risk in patients with type 2 diabetes is as high as in a non-diabetic patient after myocardial infarction, similar goals for plasma lipids are recommended, i.e. LDL-cholesterol < 100 mg/dL and triglyceride levels below 150 mg/dL (European Diabetes Association) or 200 mg/dL (American Diabetes and Heart Associations). Therefore, plasma LDL-cholesterol is normally lowered by the use of a statin.

Elevated plasma triglyceride levels can be dramatically reduced by non-pharmacological measures. If target levels are not obtained, treatment with a fibrate can be recommended. The latter is recommended because there is some recent evidence of cardiovascular risk reduction from interventional trials.

In the case presented, fibrate treatment was begun directly, because there is an increased risk of acute pancreatitis in patients with triglyceride levels above 750 mg/dL. In combined hyperlipidaemia – depending on triglyceride levels, LDL-cholesterol concentration and global risk, treatment begins either with a statin or with a fibrate. If treatment is begun with a fibrate, very often LDL-cholesterol are elevated initially because of an optimized VLDL-particle turnover. Often this elevated LDL-cholesterol level decreases again after about 6 months. Otherwise a low dose of a statin should be added. There is an absolute contraindication to combining statins with Gemfibrozil.

What did I learn from this case?

Tubero-eruptice xanthoma, typically at the extension of the arms and at the arms and the buttocks, can be the presenting complaint of high triglyceride levels.

Alterations of lipid metabolism, especially dyslipoproteinaemia, is a very early and sensitive marker of decreased insulin sensitivity and/or glucose intolerance. Therefore, dyslipoproteinaemia can be the first clinical sign of type 2 diabetes, and screening these individuals for underlying glucose intolerance by appropriate tests is recommended. It should be borne in mind that alcohol can dramatically aggravate a hypertriglyceridaemia.

Even minor reductions in body weight can lead to a dramatic increase in insulin sensitivity and thereby lowering of plasma triglycerides.

How much did this case alter my approach to the care and treatment of my patients with diabetes?

We have learnt to screen for underlying glucose intolerance in patients with dyslipoproteinaemia. The patient with type 2 diabetes is a high coronary risk patient, similar to a post-myocardial infarct patient. Therefore, classical coronary risk factors such as plasma lipids, should be treated aggressively. Type 2 diabetes is more than just a clinical state of increased blood sugar levels.

Further reading

American Diabetes Association. Clinical practice recommendations 1999. *Diabetes Care* 22 (Suppl 1): S56–S59.

Expert Panel on Detection, Evaluation, and Treatment of High Blood Cholesterol in Adults: Executive Summary of the Third Report of the National Education Program (NCEP) Expert Panel on Detection, Evaluation, and Treatment of High Blood Cholesterol in Adults (Adult Treatment Panel III). *JAMA* 2001; 185: 2486–97.

CASE 37: SEVERE HYPER-TRIGLYCERIDAEMIA IN PREGNANCY PRESENTING AS PANCREATITIS

Andrew I Pettit, James M Lawrence,
Andrew Taylor, Anthony M Robinson
and John PD Reckless

During normal pregnancy triglyceride levels rise especially during the third trimester. However, the physiological rise can be exaggerated, particularly in mothers with poorly controlled diabetes. We would like to present two cases of severe hypertriglyceridaemia in pregnancy presenting as pancreatitis.

Case one—History

The first patient presented at 28 weeks in her third pregnancy with a history of two days of intermittent, severe, gripping epigastric and chest pain aggravated by movement, inspiration and lying flat. Up to that point the pregnancy had been unremarkable and foetal movements were normal. She had no past medical history of note. Her first pregnancy had ended in a miscarriage at 12 weeks and the second had ended with spontaneous premature labour at 31 weeks, with delivery of a healthy boy weighing 1.82 kg. On initial assessment, the patient was in some distress with a sinus tachycardia of 120 beats/min and mild epigastric tenderness. When blood was drawn, it was noted to be markedly lipaemic. This was confirmed in the laboratory with triglycerides of 107.3 mmol/L and cholesterol of 34 mmol/L. The full blood count showed a neutrophil leucocytosis (WBC 16.6, neutrophils 14.5, Hb 10.0 and platelets 240). Sodium 133 mmol/L, potassium 3.7 mmol/L, creatinine 58 µmol/L, alkaline phosphatase 70 IU/L, albumin 30, globulin 25, ALT 25, and amylase 60 U/L, were normal. At this stage it was considered possible that the cause of the patient's abdominal pain was pancreatitis secondary to the gross hypertriglyceridaemia. The amylase assay was re-run in dilution but still produced a result in the normal range. Following discussion with the biochemistry laboratory, a urine sample was sent for amylase measurement in view of the possibility of the marked hypertriglyceridaemia interfering with the serum amylase assay. The urine amylase was modestly raised at 1911 IU/L (normal <960 IU/L), supporting the presumptive diagnosis. An abdominal ultrasound was also consistent with pancreatitis but, more importantly, did not show any dilatation of the biliary tree. On further examination, the patient was noted to have lipaemia retinalis but no other stigmata of hyperlipidaemia. She had no family history of a lipid disorder.

The patient was initially kept nil by mouth, and an intravenous infusion was set up. In an attempt to reduce the triglycerides, she was commenced on an infusion of 10% dextrose with 20 mmol/L KCl every 12 h, with intravenous insulin delivered at 3–4 units/h, aiming to keep the blood glucose between 4 and 7 mmol/L. The abdominal pain resolved over the first 48 h, and the triglycerides gradually fell to 19.9 mmol/L over the first week. At that stage the sliding-scale insulin was stopped, and the patient was started on a low-fat diet in conjunction with MaxEPA 5 g bid. After a further 24 h she was commenced on a basal-bolus insulin regime with 4 units Actrapid before each meal and 4 units Insulatard at night. An increased dose of MaxEPA of 10 g bid was not tolerated, inducing marked nausea. The patient was discharged home after two weeks with triglycerides of 18.8 mmol/L. On subsequent review in the antenatal clinic, her lipid profile had improved, and she had had no episodes of hypoglycaemia on insulin. Labour was induced at 38 weeks and proceeded uneventfully with delivery of a girl weighing 3.71 kg. Insulin was stopped at delivery, and lipids were re-checked 2 weeks after birth; as triglycerides were 3.9 mmol/L, the MaxEPA was stopped. At 6 weeks post-delivery, a glucose tolerance test was performed (fasting 5.3 mmol/L and 2 h post 3.9 mmol/L). The triglyceride levels off MaxEPA were 2.7 mmol/L.

Case two—History

The second patient is a woman of 24 years of age with a history over 4 years of diet-controlled diabetes, diagnosed during an admission to hospital with pancreatitis. Following her initial presentation, she gave a history of recurrent mild central abdominal pain over the next 3 years. She was admitted to hospital again 1 year later with a history over 3 days of constant, severe, central abdominal pain associated with vomiting. A clinical diagnosis of pancreatitis was made, although the serum amylase was only 225 IU/L (no urinary amylase was requested). Serum was noted to be lipaemic, and on analysis triglycerides were markedly elevated at 31 mmol/L. She responded well to iv fluids and prior to discharge was commenced on fenofibrate micro 200 mg od, increasing to 267 mg od, and MaxEPA 5 g bid. At subsequent review, her lipid profile had markedly improved (cholesterol 4.6 mmol/L, triglycerides 7.8 mmol/L, HDL 0.6 mmol/L), and she felt well. She was noted to have acanthosis nigricans, suggesting significant insulin resistance, and was commenced on metformin 500 mg bid, increasing to 1 g bid. Shortly afterwards, the patient presented in early pregnancy. Her fenofibrate micro and MaxEPA were stopped, and she was transferred from metformin to insulin therapy. At 22 weeks pregnant she was admitted to hospital

Table 1 Changes in lipid parameters and treatment over time of case 1 – baby delivered at 73 days

Day	1	2	4	6	8	12	19	29	45	63	84
Triglyceride (mmol/L)	107.3	74	34.1	23.5	21.8	17	12.7	7.9	7	7.2	3
Cholesterol (mmol/L)	34.2	34		23.5	23.5	20.9	9.8	8.2	6.1	7	7.9

Insulin and dextrose infusion (day 2–8)

with a further episode of severe abdominal pain with vomiting. A presumptive diagnosis of pancreatitis secondary to hypertriglyceridaemia (admission triglycerides 38 mmol/L) was made. She was treated with analgesia, iv fluids and insulin and gradually improved. She was reviewed in clinic 2 weeks after discharge. She was asymptomatic but with elevated lipids (cholesterol 10.3 mmol/L, triglycerides 18.7 mmol/L, HDL 1.2 mmol/L). She remained well through the rest of pregnancy and was induced at 38 weeks, delivering a healthy girl weighing 3.5 kg. Post-delivery insulin was stopped and she was restarted on metformin, MaxEPA 5 mg bid and fenofibrate micro 267 mg od. She will be kept under regular review in clinic.

Commentary

Hypertriglyceridaemia in pregnancy

In normal pregnancies triglyceride levels rise 2–3-fold in the third trimester,[1] correlating with maternal oestrogen levels. There are a number of described mutations of lipoprotein lipase[2-5] that under normal circumstances would result in normal or near-normal fasting triglycerides and would be asymptomatic. The raised oestrogen levels later in pregnancy unmask the deficiency causing the triglyceride levels to rise to dangerous levels. There have been reports of oral contraceptives containing 50 µg of oestrogen,[6] hormone replacement therapy[7] and clomiphene[8] also resulting in severely raised triglycerides and pancreatitis.

Pancreatitis in pregnancy due to raised triglycerides has not always been well recognized and has been considered a rare problem, with only 10 English language case reports between 1956 and 1990.[9] However, as more cases are recognized, other authors have identified severe hypertriglyceridaemia as the most frequent cause of pancreatitis in pregnancy.[10] Outside pregnancy estimates vary from less than 5% to at least 10% of cases of pancreatitis being associated with raised triglycerides.[11] If elevated triglycerides occur in one pregnancy, they are likely to occur in subsequent pregnancies too and, without treatment, may cause recurrent foetal loss.[12] Severe hypertriglyceridaemia of pregnancy usually becomes apparent in the third trimester but may present in the second.[1] The mortality from pancreatitis due to high triglycerides of pregnancy is significant for both mother and foetus at approximately 20%.[1]

Primary causes of severely elevated triglyceride levels are lipoprotein lipase deficiency and Apo CII deficiency.[13] Both are rare recessive conditions (each is thought to have a population frequency of 1 in 10⁶) that present in childhood with recurrent abdominal pain with or without pancreatitis. Other features include eruptive xanthomas, a cream layer on the surface of blood samples left standing, lipaemia retinalis, hepatosplenomegaly due to accumulation of triglycerides in the reticuloendothelial system and, less frequently, breathlessness and neurological sequelae. Both lipoprotein lipase deficiency and Apo CII deficiency result in accumulation of triglyceride because of reduced clearance. Lipoprotein lipase hydrolyzes triglyceride and Apo CII is a co-factor for lipoprotein lipase activation and a ligand for binding chylomicrons, very-low-density lipoproteins and low-density lipoproteins. Therefore absent Apo CII results in a functional deficiency of lipoprotein lipase. Heterozygotes for each deficiency occur with a frequency of approximately 1 in 500 in most populations. Although they have only 50% lipoprotein lipase activity, they rarely have raised triglycerides in the absence of secondary causes, such as poorly controlled diabetes, alcoholism, obesity, oestrogen therapy, hypothyroidism and nephrotic syndrome.

Pathophysiology of pancreatitis in hypertriglyceridaemia

The mechanism by which the raised triglycerides cause pancreatitis is unclear. One possible mechanism is the uptake of increased amounts of triglyceride by the pancreas, which is then broken down by pancreatic lipases to fatty acids and lysolecithin, causing chemical irritation of the pancreas.[13] Others believe that the severe hypertriglyceridaemia results in increased blood viscosity that slows blood flow, causing relative tissue hypoxia. The very high levels of substrate in close anatomical proximity to pancreatic lipases can result in activation of the lipases, causing tissue necrosis and autodigestion to ensue.

Investigation of abdominal pain in patients with hypertriglyceridaemia

Raised triglyceride levels may become apparent before pancreatitis occurs, as the patient may develop eruptive zanthomas and blood samples may be recognized as being lipaemic. If pancreatitis does occur, confirmation of it can be difficult. Triglyceride levels of such a magnitude occupy a large plasma volume and effectively dilute other solutes, classically causing pseudo-hyponatraemia, unless values are corrected for serum water, or measured by direct ion-selective electrode.[13] In both cases the serum amylase was low, which is a recognized feature of the older amylase assays in the presence of raised triglyceride levels. However, the newer enzymatic, chromogenic assays should yield accurate results despite severe hypertriglyceridaemia. According to the manufacturers, with the kynetic assay used in our laboratory (Amyl: Roche Diagnostics, Mannheim, Germany) there is no significant interference from triglycerides up to a concentration of about 30 mmol/L. To avoid missing the diagnosis of pancreatitis, urinary amylase should be checked where there is clinical suspicion and there is severe hypertriglyceridaemia. Serum lipase assay may be helpful, but very few laboratories in the UK offer the service. In case 1, it was felt that the modestly raised urinary amylase, pancreatic oedema on ultrasound, severe hypertriglyceridaemia and the clinical picture were sufficient to confirm the diagnosis. In case 2, the diagnosis was presumptive based on the presenting features and past history of recurrent pancreatitis.

177

Causes of secondary hypertriglyceridaemia should be excluded. Therefore a history of alcohol consumption should be ascertained and mean corpuscular volume (MCV) and gamma-glutamyl transferase (γGT) measured; diabetic control assessed or diabetes screened for in patients not previously known to be diabetic; thyroid function tests performed; and nephrotic syndrome excluded. If no secondary cause can be found, the underlying aetiology of raised triglyceride levels can be ascertained by measuring basal and heparin-stimulated lipoprotein lipase activity, and Apo CII levels can be assayed. Although lipoprotein lipase activity can be quantified and Apo CII measured, they are not routinely available and have not been assayed in pregnancy. Analysis of the genetic defect resulting in the reduced LPL activity is not widely available.

Treatment of pancreatitis due to hypertriglyceridaemia in pregnancy

Treatment of acute pancreatitis during pregnancy owing to raised triglyceride is generally as for any other episode of pancreatitis: fluid resuscitation, nil by mouth, analgesia, and ventilation if features of adult respiratory distress syndrome are present. Severe hypertriglyceridaemia associated with pancretitis, as assessed by Glasgow criteria, has been treated with plasmapheresis since the late 1970s[14,15] to achieve rapid reduction of triglyceride levels. More recently, there have been numerous reports of the use of plasmapheresis in pregnancy with good foetal and maternal outcomes.[1,16–20]

There are various strategies for the subsequent management of the hypertriglyceridaemia. Pancreatitis can occur with triglyceride levels >10 mmol/L and especially if >20 mmol/L. If pancreatitis has previously occured, it is much more likely to recur at similar or lower triglyceride levels. Safe levels may be achieved by restriction of dietary fat intake to 10% of the total calorie intake,[13] but this is very difficult to achieve and not well tolerated. If dietary restriction is prolonged, supplementation of the fat-soluble vitamins is required. Medium-chain triglycerides may be used as an alternative calorie source to long-chain triglycerides. Medium-chain triglycerides are absorbed directly into the portal circulation and therefore bypass chylomicron formation. Unfortunately, medium-chain triglycerides are not very palatable. Elemental diets and parenteral nutrition have both been used but tend to be reserved for cases where dietary restriction alone produces an insufficient lowering of triglycerides to safe levels (<10 mmol/L).[5,17,21] Both insulin and heparin are known to activate lipoprotein lipase, and there are case reports of both being used in pancreatitis owing to elevated triglycerides.[21,22] In diabetic patients with pancreatitis during pregnancy, it is essential to optimize their glucose control, but intravenous and subcutaneous insulin has been used in non-diabetic subjects too. Heparin will have no effect in homozygous lipoprotein lipase and Apo CII deficiency, and insulin will only help reduce triglycerides in subjects who are also diabetic or insulin resistant. Omega-

3 fish oils (MaxEPA) can be used safely in pregnancy,[22] the dose being titrated to response or to side-effects. There is reluctance to prescribe fibrates in pregnancy, but there are a few case reports of the use of gemfibrozil[1,3] and bezafibrate[21] in pregnancy with good maternal and foetal outcomes. Early delivery (38/52) is advocated by many.

After pregnancy the triglyceride levels return to normal or near-normal but, as the underlying aetiology of the raised triglycerides of pregnancy is likely to be reduced lipoprotein lipase function that is unmasked in the third trimester of pregnancy, it would be wise to advise the mother to avoid secondary causes of raised triglycerides. This would involve avoiding excess alcohol, particularly binge drinking, ensuring that diabetic patients are well controlled, and careful consideration of mode of subsequent contraception, as the oestrogen-containing oral contraceptive pill may provoke further rises in triglyceride levels. For the same reasons, later in life hormone replacement therapy would be ill advised, unless given as oestrogen patches to largely bypass first-pass hepatic removal. Adoption of a healthy lifestyle should be encouraged with particular emphasis on weight control. The issue of subsequent pregnancies is difficult, as the chances of developing severe hypertriglyceridaemia and pancreatitis are high. The risks can be minimized by adherence to very low-fat diet and regular fasting TG levels throughout pregnancy, with particular attention to the lipids from 20 weeks onwards. If levels rise above 10 mmol/L, a number of preventive strategies can be considered; parenteral nutrition[5] has been tried and MaxEPA is felt to be safe during pregnancy.

Hypertriglyceridaemia in polycystic ovarian syndrome

The occurrence of severe hypertriglyceridaemia in polycystic ovarian syndrome could be expected owing to the insulin resistance and obesity, but there is little evidence to support this supposition. There are no published data on triglyceride levels in polycystic ovarian syndrome, and only one case report of a woman with polycystic ovarian syndrome having mildly raised triglycerides,[23] who subsequently developed eruptive xanthomas when she became diabetic while also on an oestrogen-containing oral contraceptive. At a later stage the woman was also found to have a deficiency of Apo CII.

Hypertriglyceridaemia in diabetes

Severe hypertriglyceridaemia is recognized in insulin-dependent diabetes,[24] non-insulin-dependent diabetes and gestational diabetes,[21] especially when the diabetes is poorly controlled and can lead to pancreatitis. Other factors that might synergistically act to raise triglycerides levels in diabetic patients are the oral contraceptive pill, hormone replacement therapy,[7] pregnancy, obesity and protease inhibitors used in the treatment of HIV.[25]

Pancreatitis is probably also under-diagnosed in diabetic ketoacidosis. There are a number of case reports of severe hypertriglyceridaemia, pancreatitis and diabetic ketoacidosis. Nair et al.[26] prospectively studied 100 patients admitted with diabetic ketoacidosis. All patients had serum triglyceride, amylase and lipase measured, and those with triglyceride levels three times higher than normal or amylase/lipase levels greater than twice normal had ultrasound or CT imaging of the pancreas. Pancreatitis was diagnosed if pancreatic oedema was found. Using these criteria, 11 patients were found to have pancreatitis, 8 of whom had abdominal pain, 2 had no pain and 1 was comatose. The aetiology of pancreatitis was thought to be hypertriglyceridaemia in 4 patients, alcohol in 2, drugs in 1 and idiopathic in 4. Nair et al. also point out that diabetic ketoacidosis can mildly elevate serum amylase levels and that Ranson's scale tends to overestimate the severity of pancreatitis in diabetic ketoacidosis.[27] Instead of Ranson's scale, Nair et al. suggest assessing severity on the degree of pancreatic oedema found on imaging. There is only one case report of hyperosmolar non-ketotic diabetic coma or pre-coma being associated with pancreatitis,[28] and the underlying aetiology of the pancreatitis was uncertain.

The treatment of diabetic patients with pancreatitis due to severe hypertriglyceridaemia is the same as for pancreatitis in pregnancy due to severe hypertriglyceridaemia. Plasmapheresis has been successfully used in diabetic patients with acute pancreatitis,[14] and subsequent treatment has consisted of good diabetic control, dietary fat restriction and weight loss. The fibrates can reduce triglyceride levels by 50%;[29] omega-3 fish oils in small studies were found to lower triglycerides by 50%;[30] and case reports suggest that nicotinic acid can also be very effective.[31]

References

1. Perrone G, Critelli C. [Severe hypertriglyceridaemia in pregnancy. A clinical case report]. *Minerva Ginecol* 1996; **48**(12): 573–6.

2. Henderson H, Leisegang F, Hassan F, Hayden M, Marais D. A novel Glu421Lys substitution in the lipoprotein lipase gene in pregnancy-induced hypertriglyceridaemic pancreatitis. *Clin Chim Acta* 1998; **269**(1): 1 12.

3. Keilson LM, Vary CP, Sprecher DL, Renfrew R. Hyperlipidemia and pancreatitis during pregnancy in two sisters with a mutation in the lipoprotein lipase gene. *Ann Intern Med* 1996; **124**(4): 425 8.

4. Ma Y, Ooi TC, Liu MS et al. High frequency of mutations in the human lipoprotein lipase gene in pregnancy-induced chylomicronemia: possible association with apolipoprotein E2 isoform. *J Lipid Res* 1994; **35**(6): 1066–75.

5. Weinberg RB, Sitrin MD, Adkins GM, Lin CC. Treatment of hyperlipidemic

pancreatitis in pregnancy with total parenteral nutrition. *Gastroenterology* 1982; **83**(6): 1300–5.

6. Muller DP, Pavlou C, Whitelaw AG, McLintock D. The effect of pregnancy and two different contraceptive pills on serum lipids and lipoproteins in a woman with a type III hyperlipoproteinaemia pattern. *Br J Obstet Gynaecol* 1978; **85**(2): 127–33.

7. Sattar N, Jaap AJ. Hormone replacement preparations and hypertriglyceridaemia in women with NIDDM. *Diabetes Care* 1997; **20**(2): 234–5.

8. Castro MR, Nguyen TT, O'Brien T. Clomiphene-induced severe hypertriglyceridaemia and pancreatitis. *Mayo Clin Proc* 1999; **74**(11): 1125–8.

9. Nies BM, Dreiss RJ. Hyperlipidemic pancreatitis in pregnancy: a case report and review of the literature. *Am J Perinatol* 1990; **7**(2): 166–9.

10. Chang CC, Hsieh YY, Tsai HD, Yang TC, Yeh LS, Hsu TY. Acute pancreatitis in pregnancy. *Chung Hua I Hsueh Tsa Chih (Taipei)* 1998; **61**(2): 85–92.

11. Durrington PN. *Hyperlipidaemia: Diagnosis and management*. Oxford: Butterworth-Heinemann, 1995.

12. Suga S, Tamasawa N, Kinpara I et al. Identification of homozygous lipoprotein lipase gene mutation in a woman with recurrent aggravation of hypertriglyceridaemia induced by pregnancy. *J Intern Med* 1998; **243**(4): 317–21.

13. Mahley RW, Weisgraber KH, Farese RV jr. Disorders of lipid metabolism. In: Wilson JD, Foster DW, Kronenberg HM, Larsen PR (eds). *Williams Textbook of Endocrinology* 9th edn. Philadelphia: Saunders, 1998: chapter 23.

14. Betteridge DJ, Bakowski M, Taylor KG et al. Treatment of severe diabetic hypertriglyceridaemia by plasma exchange. *Lancet* 1978; **1**: 1368.

15. Kollef MH, McCormack MT, Caras WE, Reddy VV, Bacon D. The fat overload syndrome: successful treatment with plasma exchange. *Ann Intern Med* 1990; **112**: 545–6.

16. Achard JM, Westeel PF, Moriniere P, Lalau JD, de Cagny B, Fournier A. Pancreatitis related to severe acute hypertriglyceridaemia during pregnancy: treatment with lipoprotein apheresis. *Intensive Care Med* 1991; **17**(4): 236–7.

17. Hsia SH, Connelly PW, Hegele RA. Successful outcome in severe pregnancy-associated hyperlipemia: a case report and literature review. *Am J Med Sci* 1995; **309**(4): 213–18.

18. Swoboda K, Derfler K, Koppensteiner R et al. Extracorporeal lipid elimination for treatment of gestational hyperlipidemic pancreatitis. *Gastroenterology* 1993; **104**(5): 1527–31.

19. Saravanan P, Blumenthal S, Anderson C, Stein R, Berkelhammer C. Plasma exchange for dramatic gestational hyperlipidemic pancreatitis. *J Clin Gastroenterol* 1996; **22**(4): 295–8.

20. Yamauchi H, Sunamura M, Takeda K, Suzuki T, Itoh K, Miyagawa K. Hyperlipidemia and pregnancy associated pancreatitis with reference to plasma exchange as a therapeutic intervention. *Tohoku J Exp Med* 1986; **148**(2): 197–205.

21. Bar-David J, Mazor M, Leiberman JR, Ielig I, Maislos M. Gestational diabetes complicated by severe hypertriglyceridaemia and acute pancreatitis. *Arch Gynecol Obstet* 1996; **258**(2): 101–4.

22. Henzen C, Rock M, Schnieper C, Heer K. [Heparin and insulin in the treatment of acute hypertriglyceridaemia-induced pancreatitis]. *Schweiz Med Wochenschr* 1999; **129**(35): 1242–8.

23. Thomas DJ, Stocks J, Galton DJ, Besser GM. Hypertriglyceridaemia and diabetes mellitus: cause or effect? *Diabet Med* 1988; **5**(1): 85–6.

24. Krauss RM, Levy AG. Subclinical chronic pancreatitis in type I hyperlipoproteinemia. *Am J Med* 1977; **62**: 144–9.

25. Meyer L, Rabaud C, Ziegler O, May T, Drouin P. Protease inhibitors, diabetes mellitus and blood lipids. *Diabetes Metab* 1998; **24**(6): 547–9.

26. Nair S, Yadav D, Pitchumoni CS. Association of diabetic ketoacidosis and acute pancreatitis: observations in 100 consecutive episodes of DKA. *Am J Gastroenterol* 2000; **95**(10): 2795–800.

27. Ranson JH, Rifkind KM, Roses DF, Fink SD, Eng K, Spencer J. Prognostic signs and the role of operative management in acute pancreatitis. *Surg Gynecol Obstet* 1974; **139**: 69–81.

28. Randeva HS, Bolodeoku J, Mikhailidis DP et al. Elevated serum creatine kinase activity in a patient with acute pancreatitis. *Int J Clin Pract* 1999; **53**: 482–3.

29. Garg A, Grundy SM. Gemfibrozil alone and in combination with lovastatin for treatment of hypertriglyceridaemia in NIDDM. *Diabetes* 1989; **38**(3): 364–72.

30. Richter WO, Jacob BG, Ritter MM, Schwandt P. Treatment of primary chylomicronemia due to familial hypertriglyceridaemia by omega-3 fatty acids. *Metabolism* 1992; **41**(10): 1100–5.

31. Smith SR. Severe hypertriglyceridaemia responding to insulin and nicotinic acid therapy. *Postgrad Med J* 1981; **57**(670): 511–15.

CASE 38: A DIAGNOSIS OF CELLULITIS IN A NEUROISCHAEMIC FOOT

Michael Edmonds

History

A 48-year-old patient with insulin-dependent diabetes for 20 years presented with a 1-week history of malaise and high blood glucose and a 2-day history of discomfort and redness of the right foot. There was no history of trauma.

He was known to have peripheral neuropathy, previously complicated by foot ulceration. He also had background retinopathy and proteinuria.

Examination and investigations

The patient had an area of erythema over the dorsum and both medial and lateral aspects of the right foot, which was also oedematous. There was no break in the skin.

Body temperature was 39.2°C, pulse 104 regular, foot pulses absent, chest clear, abdomen normal, diminished sensation to vibration and light touch in a stocking distribution in the feet and lower legs, absent ankle jerks.

Haemoglobin 11.4 g/dL, white blood count 17,300 10(9)/L, platelets 69010(9)/L, ESR 105, creatinine 82. HbA1 13%, glucose 18.6 mmol/L.

X-ray of the right foot was normal.

Blood cultures: no growth. There was no open lesion from which to take a swab. Urine protein was 535 mg in 24 hours.

Doppler studies in both legs showed a very high ankle–brachial systolic pressure ratio (> 1.5), indicative of calcification. The foot artery waveforms were damped, indicating reduced blood flow.

Diagnosis

A clinical diagnosis of cellulitis in a neuroischaemic foot was made. The other much less likely diagnosis was an acute-onset Charcot foot. However, it is unusual for a Charcot foot to be associated with such a high body temperature and chills, which is much more suggestive of sepsis.

Treatment and outcome

The patient was treated with quadruple intravenous antibiotic therapy, amoxycillin 500 mg tds, flucloxacillin 500 mg qds, metronidazole 500 mg tds and ceftazidime 1 g tds, to provide a broad-spectrum cover.[1] The patient was commenced on sliding scale intravenous insulin.

By the next day, body temperature had fallen to 37.2°C (Figure 1) but there was no improvement in the cellulitis. There were spikes of fever on the evening of the second and third days. The area of cellulitis did not regress but there was no evidence of a collection of pus. A surgical opinion was obtained and it confirmed that there was no indication for surgery.

On the fourth day of the admission the patient was still pyrexial. He also had a rigor. The ceftazidime was withdrawn and intravenous gentamicin 80 mg tds was started. The most common organism isolated from diabetic foot infections is *Staphylococcus aureus* and gentamicin is active against *Staph. aureus* as well as providing gram-negative cover.

On the fifth day, the patient remained pyrexial and a patch of purplish discolouration was noted within the area of erythema (Figure 2). In very severe cases of cellulitis, bluish-purplish discolouration of the skin indicates subcutaneous necrosis. The patient underwent surgical debridement of the area of discolouration. Subcutaneous necrosis and pus were noted. There was a wide

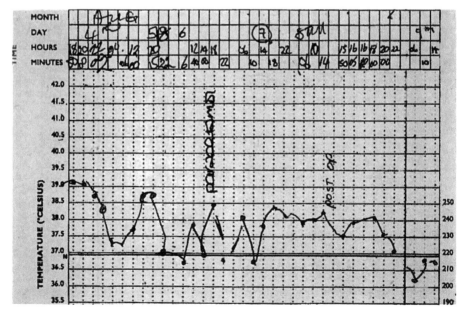

Figure 1 *Patient's temperature chart.*

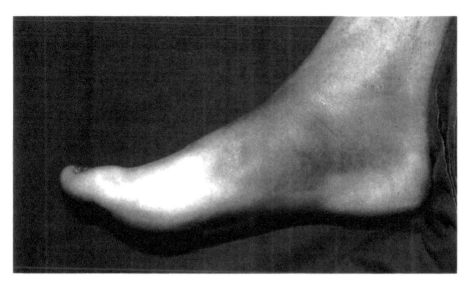

Figure 2 *Area of erythema on patient's foot.*

excision of an ellipse of skin and subcutaneous tissue 1.3 × 1.0 × 0.3 cm in depth. Histology showed fibrous connective tissue, fat and necrotic debris showing extensive necrosis with haemorrhage.

Tissue and pus were sent for culture; both grew *Staph. aureus*. Antibiotic therapy specifically for *Staph. aureus* was prescribed including rifampicin, flucloxacillin and gentamicin. The patient's temperature resolved within 2 days.

In view of the Doppler studies, the patient underwent a transfemoral angiogram. This showed a 90% stenosis just distal to the origin of the right posterior tibial artery with a diffusely diseased common femoral artery. The patient underwent angioplasty of the posterior tibial artery, 10 days after the surgical debridement. Finally, a split skin graft was applied to the wound.

Commentary

The patient had been feeling generally unwell with malaise and poor diabetic control. These may be the first signs of a foot infection. The patient may have thought that he had flu at this stage but there were no symptoms in the infected foot.

The patient complained of discomfort in his foot. In the presence of neuropathy, lesions of the foot may be painless. However, new pain may indicate infection.

Body temperature on admission was 39.2°C. However, 50% of patients with diabetic foot infections do not develop a fever.[2,3] When they do, it is a good parameter, by which response to treatment can be judged.

In very severe cases of cellulitis, bluish-purplish discolouration of the skin indicates subcutaneous necrosis. This is caused by increased metabolic demands of infection and a reduction of blood flow to the skin secondary to a septic vasculitis of the cutaneous circulation. Blue discolouration can occur in both the neuropathic and also the neuroischaemic foot, and in the neuroischaemic foot it must not be automatically attributed to worsening ischaemia of the leg arteries. At this point the tissue is not frankly necrotic but has started to break down and liquefy. It is best for this tissue to be removed operatively.

In the management of the infected diabetic foot, the definite indications for urgent surgical intervention are purplish discolouration of the skin including subcutaneous necrosis, a large area of infected sloughy tissue, localized fluctuation and crepitus with gas in the soft tissues on X-ray. All infections cannot simply be treated with intravenous antibiotics. There may be a need for surgical debridement. This is an important decision in the care of the patient and needs to be jointly carried out in the multidisciplinary foot care team. Daily inspection of the foot is mandatory. If fever does not resolve, then further intervention is necessary.

Learning points

- Infected diabetic feet with severe cellulitis need daily inspection and assessment.
- The development of bluish-purplish discolouration of the skin indicates subcutaneous necrosis. This needs urgent surgical debridement and the tissue removed should be sent for culture. It is then possible to target the antibiotic therapy towards the organisms responsible for the infection, having started with broad-spectrum antibiotic therapy.
- The microbiology of the diabetic foot is unique. Infection can be caused by gram-positive, gram-negative and anaerobic bacteria, singly or in combination. Antibiotics alone do not treat foot infections. However, at initial presentation, it is important to prescribe a wide spectrum of antibiotics because it is impossible to predict the organisms from the clinical appearance. If the patient undergoes operative debridement, then deep tissue should also be sent for culture.
- It is important to explore the possibility of revascularization in the infected neuroischaemic foot. Improvement of perfusion will not only help to control infection but will also promote healing of wounds if operative debridement is necessary.
- Angiography should be carried out to detect the presence of stenoses or occlusions, which may be amenable to angioplasty or bypass. Duplex angiography may initially be carried out, followed by angioplasty. Alternatively, transfemoral angiography can be performed as the initial procedure.

- Angioplasty is indicated in the treatment of single or multiple stenoses or short segment occlusions of < 10 cm. If angioplasty is not possible because of long arterial occlusions, bypass should be considered.

How much did this alter my approach to the care and treatment of my patients with diabetes?

Infection in the diabetic foot is a medical emergency and patients need close daily supervision with combined input from medical and surgical teams.

References

1. Edmonds ME, Foster AVM. *Managing the Diabetic Foot*. Oxford: Blackwell Science, 2000.

2. Eneroth M, Apelqvist J, Stenstrom A. Clinical characteristics and outcome in 223 diabetic patients with deep foot infections. *Foot Ankle Int* 1997; 18: 716–22.

3. Armstrong DG, Lavery LA, Sariaya M, Ashry H. Leukocytosis is a poor indicator of acute osteomyelitis of the foot in diabetes mellitus. *J Foot Ankle Surg* 1996; 4: 280–3.

Case 39: Poor diabetic control, weight loss and pain in the thighs

Poonam Bhalla and Gareth Williams

History

TB was diagnosed with insulin-dependent diabetes mellitus (IDDM) at the age of 16 years and initially treated with twice-daily Monotard and Actrapid. From the outset, her diabetic control was erratic, with recurrent episodes of ketoacidosis and weight loss (Figure 1). Hospital admissions were frequent and necessitated time off school while she was studying for A' levels (six admissions totalling 10 weeks as an inpatient).

Aged 21, she was admitted to hospital following a period of particularly poor control, complaining of excruciating thigh pain and depressive symptoms. She had bilateral quadriceps wasting, thigh weakness and absent ankle reflexes; diabetic

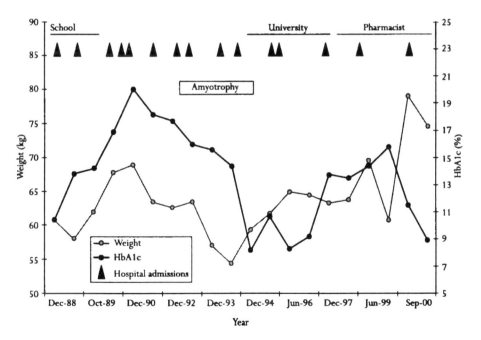

Figure 1 *Changes in TB's weight and glycated haemoglobin (HbA1c) concentration. Hospital admissions and the period of painful amyotrophy are also shown.*

amyotrophy was diagnosed. Diabetic control was improved and she was given amitriptyline; her pain and depression improved gradually over 4–6 months.

While training as a pharmacist, TB continued to live at home with her parents. She found the pharmacy course work stressful and her depression returned. Her relationship with her mother, always stormy, deteriorated further. It transpired that she was afraid of inheriting her mother's obesity. At the time, her body mass index (BMI) was 23 kg/m². At this point she admitted to some suicidal ideation and, for the first time, to bingeing on food and omitting insulin for up to 3 days at a time to try to control her weight. TB felt unsupported and unable to cope, and could see no way forward. With the help of the diabetes specialist nurse and further treatment with amitriptyline, her confidence (but not her diabetic control) improved. Two years later she graduated and began work as a pharmacist. She had lost 2 kg in weight and her BMI was 22.6 kg/m².

The next 12 months were erratic. She initially gained 6 kg, then became distressed about her appearance and lost 9 kg over 7 months, to a BMI of 21.5 kg/m². Her self-reported blood glucose values were mostly 7–12 mmol/L, but HbA1c was consistently 14–16%, despite an optimized twice-daily Humalog and Humulin I regimen. Because of recurrent depression, she was prescribed sertraline.

TB defaulted from follow-up until, a year later, she suffered a respiratory arrest after an emergency appendicectomy; this scared her into taking stock of her life and health. She talked openly about her previously poor compliance and her omission of both insulin and antidepressants. She started a new job, with which she was much happier, and her family relationships (particularly with her mother) improved. For the first time, she accepted counselling with a clinical psychologist and a dietician, to whom she admitted feelings of ugliness, worthlessness and revulsion at her weight.

Currently, she has discontinued her follow-up with the clinical psychologist but still sees the dietician and diabetes specialist nurse. She recently moved into her own house and feels a sense of independence and, for the first time appears to have accepted that diabetes is a part of her life. Her BMI is stable at 28 kg/m².

Commentary

TB illustrates the roller-coaster of emotions, body image conflict and poor glycaemic control faced by a small but significant group of type 1 diabetic patients. Their lives are dominated by episodes of ketoacidosis and/or hypoglycaemia, often frequent and at first sight, inexplicable.

There were few clues as to why a bright young girl should have such poor diabetic control. Subsequently it became clear that she was depressed and afraid of gaining weight. Her deliberate omission of insulin may have had two motives: firstly, a form of denial of the disease and secondly, to lose weight. However, this

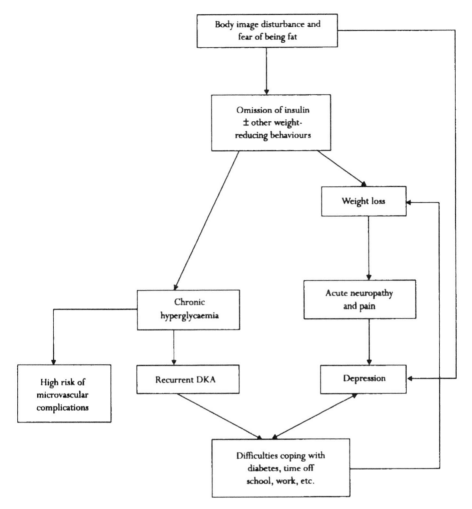

Figure 2 *The vicious circle generated by the fear of becoming obese.*

behaviour effectively locked her in the vicious circle illustrated in Figure 2, and has proved a dangerous tightrope to walk: she has already paid the price of poor diabetic control through acute neuropathy (amyotrophy), recurrent diabetic ketoacidosis (DKA) and much time spent in hospital.

Adaptation to a lifelong illness such as diabetes is not easy and often engenders emotional reactions akin to grief, over the loss of health and lifestyle. Maladaptation, where the process of learning to cope is incomplete or prolonged, is apparently commoner in young patients or those with complications of the illness. Disbelief or denial is often followed by anger (which may involve neglect of self-care) and ultimately depression, once realization of the long-term nature of the illness has dawned. Significant depression and/or anxiety probably affect up to

50% of poorly controlled young diabetic patients,[1] some of whom display clear self-destructive behaviour with serious suicidal attempts.[2]

Disturbances of body image and eating disorders have been recognized increasingly among diabetic patients, and may explain why young females generally have poorer glycaemic control[3] and more hospital admissions[4] than their male counterparts. Eating disorders were first reported in association with diabetes in three cases described in 1980,[5] and subsequent work has indicated that this is not merely a chance relationship.[6,7] There is a definite overlap between diabetic patients with eating disorders and the subgroup with 'brittle' (chronically unstable) diabetes, that consists largely of young women.[8] Insulin therapy is associated with weight gain due to its anabolic effects and many patients, especially young women, find the change in body image frightening,[9] just at a time in life when young people become acutely aware of the social and cultural pressures towards slimness. This, coupled with a desire for independence and not wanting to be different from one's peers, can easily spiral into a cycle of internal and external conflict and low self-esteem, with worsening of body-image disturbances and their physical and psychological consequences. An obvious (but erroneous) way to break out of this cycle is to take less insulin. Not surprisingly, these patients generally have poor glycaemic control[10] with constantly high HbA1c level.[11] Diabetic patients with anorexia nervosa may reduce their carbohydrate intake and insulin dosage in tandem, to avoid extreme glycaemic swings.[12] Those with bulimia may cover a food binge by temporarily increasing their insulin, which can rapidly lead to obesity. Some patients employ other well-known strategies such as self-induced vomiting or abuse of laxatives or diuretics.

There is a higher than usual incidence of early-onset microvascular complications (especially retinopathy) in diabetic patients with eating disorders.[5,7] Amyotrophy, an acute reversible mononeuropathy of the femoral nerve, is an acute neuropathic syndrome specific to diabetes mellitus. It was first described by Garland in the 1950's[13] and tends to follow severe weight loss due to periods of uncontrolled hyperglycaemia[14] or anorexia nervosa. Possible mechanisms include the metabolic effects of hyperglycaemia, a fall in circulating insulin or other growth factors, or haemodynamic changes within the nerve. Pain with or without thigh wasting is the cardinal feature[15] and weight loss may be so striking that it meets Ellenberg's description of 'neuropathic cachexia'.[16] Pain is typically neurogenic (lancinating, electric shock sensations or burning) and may be so severe that patients are driven to contemplate suicide; poor-quality sleep and depression are common accompaniments. The pain may respond to tricyclic agents; the pain and the muscle weakness and wasting tend to resolve spontaneously, but often over many months.

TB's problems were and still are a challenge to her family and her diabetes team. The advice and input of many specialists is needed, including the diabetes nurse, dietician, clinical psychologist, and where appropriate, psychiatrist. Persuading patients to accept these interventions is often difficult, especially for those trying to attend college, hold down a job or run a home. A team approach to care, from as early on as possible, serves the patient best. Ideally, a full-time clinical psychologist should be part of the diabetes team's multi-professional 'package', with easy referral pathways and enough time to see these patients as often and as intensively as they may need. Meltzer et al[17] suggest that the Eating Disorders Inventory (EDI) Bulimia subscale could be used in diabetic clinics to identify adolescents whose eating patterns are likely to compromise their glycaemic control. When worrying emotional and behavioural symptoms are noticed, appropriate members of the team can become more personally involved with the needs of each individual. An open and sympathetic discussion about why insulin therapy is needed often helps, and the patient should be asked what type of insulin regimen they would be prepared to follow. This may not be as intensive or as effective as the diabetes team would prefer, but confronting the patient about her 'non-compliance' or threatening them with the prospects of ketoacidosis or going blind are unlikely to improve an already difficult situation. These issues will never be easy to resolve, but education coupled with empathic discussion can go a long way towards preventing the multiple complex factors spiralling out of control.

What does the future hold for TB? Now aged 29, she has already suffered significant complications of non-compliance; yet she does not wish to see a psychologist and her body image disturbance remains a concern. Statistically she has a higher risk of death, and of microvascular and pregnancy complications and a poorer quality of life[18] than patients with more stable diabetes. Realistically, all we can hope to achieve is to keep supporting her as best we can, both medically and psychologically, until she is ready to live with her diabetes, and her shape.

References

1. Orr DP, Golden MP, Myers G, Marrero DG. Characteristics of adolescents with poorly controlled diabetes referred to a tertiary care centre. *Diabetes Care* 1983; 6: 170–5.

2. Stearn S. Self-destructive behaviour in young patients with diabetes mellitus. *Diabetes* 1959; 8: 379–82.

3. Jones RB, Johnston DI, Allison SP, Peacock I, Hosking DJ, Tattersall RB. Haemoglobin A1c concentrations in men and women with diabetes. *BMJ* 1984; 289: 1381.

4. Williams DRR. Hospital admissions of diabetic patients: information from Hospital Activity Analysis. *Diabetic Med* 1985; 2: 27–32.

5. Fairburn CG, Steel JM. Anorexia nervosa in diabetes mellitus. *BMJ* 1980; 280: 1167–8.

6. Rolan OM, Bhanji S. Anorexia nervosa occurring in patients with diabetes mellitus. *Postgrad Med J* 1982; 58: 354–6.

7. Powers PS, Malone I, Duncan JA. Anorexia nervosa and diabetes mellitus. *J Clin Psychiatry* 1983; **44**: 133–5.

8. Williams G, Gill GV. Eating disorders and diabetic complications. *N Engl J Med* 1997; **336**: 1905–6.

9. Steel JM, Lloyd GG, Young RJ, MacIntyre CC. Changes in eating attitudes during the first year of treatment of diabetes. *J Psychosom Res* 1990; **34**: 313–18.

10. Hillard JR, Hillard PJA. Bulimia, anorexia nervosa and diabetes. Deadly combinations. *Psychiatr Clin North Am* 1984; **7**: 367–79.

11. Rosmark B, Berne C, Holmgren S, Lago C, Renholm G, Sohlberg S. Eating disorders in patients with insulin-dependent diabetes mellitus. *J Clin Psychiatry* 1986; **47**: 547–50.

12. Biggs MM, Basco MR, Patterson G, Raskin P. Insulin withholding for weight control in women with diabetes. *Diabetes Care* 1994; **17**: 1186–9.

13. Garland H. Diabetic amyotrophy. *BMJ* 1955; **2**: 1287–90.

14. Archer AG, Watkins PJ, Thomas PK, Sharma AK, Payan J. The natural history of acute painful diabetic neuropathy. *J Neurol Neurosurg Psychiatry* 1983; **46**: 491–9.

15. Coppack SW, Watkins PJ. The natural history of femoral neuropathy. *Q J Med* 1991; **79**: 307–13.

16. Ellenberg M. Diabetic neuropathic cachexia. *Diabetes* 1974; **17**: 1178–85.

17. Meltzer LJ, Johnson SB, Prine JM, Banks RA, Desrosiers PM, Silverstein JM. Disordered eating, body mass and glycaemic control in adolescents with type 1 diabetes. *Diabetes Care* 2001; **24**: 678–82.

18. Kent LA, Gill GV, Williams G. Mortality and outcome of patients with brittle diabetes and recurrent ketoacidosis. *Lancet* 1994; **344**: 778–81.

CASE 40: DIABETIC PROXIMAL MOTOR NEUROPATHY: DOES IT RECUR?

Peter J Watkins

Introduction

Neuropathic leg pain experienced by diabetic patients with proximal motor neuropathy* causes misery not only because of pain and disability from concomitant muscle wasting, but there is also considerable anxiety with regard to the potential for future invalidism, and the fear of possible amputation. These fears are made worse by delays in establishing the correct diagnosis, with frequent referrals to rheumatologists or other specialists before the condition is recognized. Confidence is only restored when the nature of the condition is explained to patients, accompanied by an understanding of the excellent prognosis. The vital question then is 'will it recur'?

The patients presented in this commentary are unusual because of late recurrences in the contralateral leg. The patterns of onset and resolution, and recurrence and resolution, are bizarre and their sequence and implications are discussed.

History

The patient was 41 years old when he developed type 2 diabetes. A conscientious and intelligent man, he took good care both of his health in general and his diabetes in particular. He was without complications of diabetes after 30 years and enjoying good health when, aged 71 years, he developed pain in his left thigh. The description of his pain together with some wasting of thigh muscles, absence of his knee reflex and absence of clinical distal neuropathy were compatible with the diagnosis of proximal motor neuropathy. He was miserable because of the pain, but stoical and reassured by understanding that the diagnosis had a favourable prognosis. Four months after the onset, the pain had resolved, by 10 months he was asymptomatic, and the left knee reflex was recovering and weakly responsive with reinforcement.

---

*Confusion exists regarding the correct name for this condition. It was originally described by Garland and Taverner as diabetic myelopathy;[1] and the terms diabetic femoral neuropathy or amyotrophy are often used by diabetes physicians. However, neurologists also use the term lumbosacral plexopathy, but prefer the designation proximal motor neuropathy – which is the description used here.

Two years after the onset of the first episode he developed identical symptoms in his right thigh. By this time the left knee reflex had fully recovered, while the right knee reflex disappeared. The sequence of events was identical to the first episode, and 6 months after the onset, symptoms had again resolved, and both knee reflexes were restored to normal. The chronology of events is shown in Table 1.

Table 1   Case description

| Age (years) | Description | Knee jerk* | | Time (months) |
		Right	Left	
41	Type 2 diabetes (uncomplicated)	+	+	
71	Left thigh pain/weakness	+	0	0
	Pain resolved			4
	Asymptomatic	+	±	10
73	Right thigh pain/weakness	+	+	0
		0	+	3
	Pain resolved	0	+	5
74		+	+	6

The patient had no retinopathy or albuminuria.
*Knee jerk, ± = present on reinforcement only.

The patient remained reasonably healthy thereafter, developing some hypertension and claudication in his later years and dying at the age of 84 years. He never developed any notable diabetic complications, showing merely a minimal retinopathy in one eye at the age of 80 years.

Postscript

I have known very few patients who developed typical features of proximal motor neuropathy on the contralateral side 2–3 years after the first episode. Details of two further patients are shown in Table 2. They all had type 2 diabetes, were in their seventies (two men, one woman) and otherwise without diabetic

Table 2   Recurring femoral neuropathy

| Diabetes mellitus | Age at diagnosis of diabetes (years) | Age at episode | | Age at death (years) |
		1	2	
Type 2	74	75 (right)	77 (left)	80
Type 2	65	71 (right)	74 (left)	80

Diabetes was uncomplicated at onset of neuropathy.

complications. The course of their disorder was almost identical to that of the patient described above, and they all died in their eighties, several years after recovery from the second episode.

Commentary

Proximal motor neuropathy is a highly distinctive condition with a relatively rapid onset followed by virtually complete recovery after some months, with a very low risk of recurrence. It is quite unlike the gradual onset and insidious progression of the conventional long-term complications of diabetes, including symmetrical distal neuropathy, retinopathy and nephropathy, and it is not associated with them.[2] Other distinctive features are its predilection for older type 2 diabetic men[3] and indeed in as many as one third of cases it represents the presentation of the diabetes itself.[4] These are also features of other focal and multifocal asymmetrical neuropathies.[3] The pattern of the thigh pain is that of an unremitting burning sensation, often with paraesthesiae and shooting pains, and almost always including allodynia resulting in exquisite discomfort on contact with clothes and bedclothes. Sensory defects are otherwise minor, but the weakness of knee extensors and hip flexors (and occasionally the antero-lateral muscles of the lower leg) can cause major disability with collapses at the knee leading to falls. Distal sensory neuropathy is often absent, so that the apparent paradox of an absent knee reflex and intact ankle reflex is quite common.

Spontaneous full recovery is the rule in the majority of patients. Pain usually resolves in 6–12 months, the remaining discomfort disappearing after 1–3 years, leaving some patients with relatively minor sensory symptoms.[4] The knee reflex is restored in about half the patients within 3 years. Minor wasting of thigh muscles persists in some patients, but serious disability is relatively uncommon[5–7] and of our own 27 patients only 5 described limitations on walking or climbing stairs.

In our own experience of 27 patients with proximal motor neuropathy reviewed 1–14 years after the initial episode, there was only one recurrence on the same side 11 years after the first event.[4] Development of proximal motor neuropathy on the contralateral side is not rare, normally occurring within a few weeks of the first episode.[1,4,6] Late recurrences on the contralateral side are extremely rare,[1,4,8] and I have seen very few such events during 30 years of practice: three of them are shown in Table 36.2. In this situation, both patient and doctor are astonished at the precise repetition of the events experienced during the original episode. A review of 105 patients with diabetic polyradiculopathy from the Mayo Clinic also describes late recurrences in 19% of patients, usually occurring at a different site, but it is not clear how many of these referred to proximal motor neuropathy.

The cause of proximal motor neuropathy is not known. Evidence for local ischaemic changes exists with or without microinfarcts, and in some instances,[3]

197

perivascular, perineurial and subperineurial inflammatory infiltrates have been described, suggestive of an immunological process,[9] leading to the use of immunosuppression in the treatment of a few cases. Yet these patients do not have any features of systemic disease or widespread vasculitis, and many of them do not have any of the microvascular complications of diabetes either. Describing the natural history of the disease has thrown no light on the nature of the pathology, and the reason for the contralateral recurrence of this very focal disorder years after its first appearance, linked to an absence of recurrence of the same side, remains quite obscure.

What did I learn from this case?

What I have learnt from the study of these distressing cases is the importance of establishing a correct diagnosis as soon as possible and presenting the patients with the favourable prognosis which enables them to face with confidence both their protracted convalescence and recovery. They are further reassured that if the opposite side remains unaffected after some weeks, the risk of later recurrence is very rare, and on the same side almost non-existent. These reassurances play an important part in the clinical management of very distressed people who during the early days of the disease may find it hard to believe that they will not be permanently disabled.

References

1. Garland HT, Taverner D. Diabetic myelopathy. *BMJ* 1953; 1: 1405–8.

2. Watkins PJ. Clinical observations and experiments in diabetic neuropathy. *Diabetologia* 1992; 35: 2–11.

3. Said G, Thomas PK. Proximal diabetic neuropathy. In: Dyck PJ, Thomas PK, eds. *Diabetic Neuropathy*, 2nd edn. Philadelphia: WB Saunders, 1999: 474–80.

4. Coppack SW, Watkins PJ. The natural history of diabetic femoral neuropathy. *Q J Med* 1991; 79: 307–13.

5. Casey EB, Harrison MJG. Diabetic amyotrophy: a follow-up study. *BMJ* 1972; 1: 656–9.

6. Root HF, Rogers MH. Diabetic neuritis with paralysis. *N Engl J Med* 1930; 202: 1049–53.

7. Fry IK, Harwick C, Stott GW. Diabetic neuropathy: a survey and follow-up of 66 cases. *Guys Hosp Rep* 1962; 3: 113.

8. Bastron JA, Thomas JE. Diabetic polyradiculopathy. *Mayo Clin Proc* 1981; 56: 725–32.

9. Llewelyn JG, Thomas PK, King RMM. Epineurial microvasculitis in proximal diabetic neuropathy. *J Neurol* 1998; 245: 159–65.

CASE 41: A CASE OF DIABETIC FOOT ULCER

John R Turtle and P Jean Ho

History

Mr S was a 43-year-old clerical worker who was referred to the High Risk Foot Service of a Diabetes Centre at a tertiary hospital. He had had a non-healing ulcer on the plantar aspect of his left foot, underneath the head of the 5th metatarsal, for the past 18 months. Treatment had included several episodes of hospitalization with surgical interventions on the ulcer. Six weeks before he was seen, he developed another ulcer on the same foot beneath the 2nd metatarsal head, after attempts were made to reduce pressure around the first ulcer with an orthosis.

He had a 15-year history of type 2 diabetes and had been treated with maximal doses of gliclazide and metformin for the past 8 years. He had been commenced on insulin but had stopped it himself because of weight gain. For at least 2 years, glycaemic control had been poor with HbA1c values of 11.1–13.4% and symptoms of hyperglycaemia. His diet was high in fat. His job was largely sedentary and he rarely did any physical exercise.

He had long-standing paraesthesia affecting his feet and toes bilaterally. There was no previous history of foot ulcers. He denied any claudication or rest pain.

Other chronic diabetic complications included microalbuminuria and minimal non-proliferative diabetic retinopathy. He was on medication for hypertension and hypercholesterolaemia.

Examination and investigations

BMI 30.0 kg/m^2, BP 138/85 mmHg. HbA1c 12.9% (normal range 3.0–6.0%), random blood glucose 12.3 mM.

The patient was wearing open-heel sandals. His feet were dry and callused with cracked heels. The toes were clawed. On the sole of the left foot underneath the 5th metatarsal head was a 10-mm diameter punched-out ulcer. The ulcer was surrounded by a localized area of callus, redness, heat and swelling. Underneath the left 2nd metatarsal head was a smaller ulcer of similar appearance, with local inflammation (Figure 1). The skin immediately adjacent to the larger ulcer was 6.7°C warmer than the corresponding area on the right foot.

He could not feel the 10-g Semmes–Weinstein monofilament on the soles. Vibration sense was tested at the base of the medial two proximal phalanges on

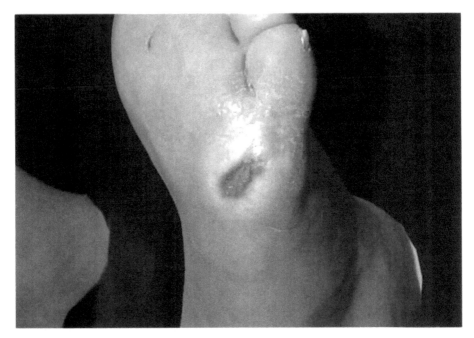

Figure 1 *Diabetic foot ulcer.*

the dorsum of each foot by biothesiometry. The patient did not feel any vibration at 50 V bilaterally. Ankle reflexes were absent. The skin colour of the feet suggested normal perfusion. The dorsalis pedis and posterior tibial pulses were palpable.

Swabs of the ulcer underneath the 5th metatarsal head grew profuse *Proteus* species and enterococci. X-ray of the left foot showed no evidence of osteomyelitis.

Diagnosis

The ulcers were clearly neuropathic and infected locally. The underlying neuropathy had caused significant sensory loss and motor dysfunction leading to clawed toes, increasing pressure underneath the metatarsal heads, and ulceration.

Treatment and outcome

Felt deflections were used to relieve pressure off the ulcer and lyofoam dressing was used. The patient was seen weekly. His partner was taught how to attend to his dressings. Callus surrounding the ulcers was debrided. He was advised to reduce the amount of walking and weight-bearing as much as possible. He was given dicloxacillin until the ulcers were healed.

In order to improve his glycaemic control and to promote wound healing Mixtard 30/70 twice a day was commenced and the dosage was titrated weekly against blood sugar levels. His oral hypoglycaemic agents were continued at maximal dosage, to enable a smaller dose of insulin to be used and this limit any weight gain associated with commencement of insulin. He was seen by the dietician and diabetes educator.

At 8 weeks both ulcers had healed. He was due to return to his local podiatrist for continued felt padding until his footwear was ready, when the ulcer under the 5th metatarsal head recurred at 9 weeks, several days after the patient did some dancing. The ulcer did not appear to be infected. It was felt that the prominence of the metatarsals and severe digital clawing were significant factors for the recurrence. Felt deflections were reapplied to relieve pressure off the ulcer. A weight-bearing X-ray was performed to better assess the bony deformity in preparation for possible surgery. An orthopaedic foot and ankle surgeon was consulted. It was thought that a further trial of felt deflections and antibiotics was worthwhile. If the ulcer did not heal despite the orthotics then forefoot reconstruction would be performed. This would involve excision arthroplasty of his 2nd to 5th metatarsal heads. It was planned to reassess the situation in 2 months time.

Commentary

Foot problems are one of the commonest problems in patients with diabetes. Patients who present with ulceration require urgent treatment of the ulcer and coexistent infection.

The treatments required for ulceration due to neuropathy and peripheral vascular disease are quite different; therefore it is necessary to distinguish these types. In this patient, the ulcers were clearly neuropathic as he could not feel the monofilament and his biothesiometer readings were high. The presence or absence of pain is not a major factor in determining the risk of neuropathic ulceration.

In most cases, inspection and palpation are adequate to assess vascular ulceration. Arterial Doppler ultrasound is used to assess the severity of peripheral vascular disease when foot pulses are very weak or impalpable, or as a pre-operative assessment of vascular supply. The ratio of the systolic blood pressure at the dorsalis pedis or tibialis posterior arteries to that at the brachial artery is called the ankle brachial index (ABI). As a guide, an ABI of 0.9–1.2 indicates that the risk of vascular foot ulceration is small. An ABI of 0.6–0.9 indicates a moderate risk and depends on the presence of other risk factors. An ABI of < 0.6 indicates a very high risk.

When there are signs of infection in the ulcer, one must distinguish between localized and generalized foot infection. In localized foot infection, signs of inflammation are confined to the area surrounding the ulcer. In contrast, in generalized foot infection, the whole foot is hot.

All patients with foot ulcers should have an X-ray to identify any underlying osteomyelitis, which would then require more intensive antimicrobial therapy. An X-ray may also locate foreign bodies which have punctured the insensate foot and remained in the soft tissue. Weight-bearing X-rays are particularly important in assessing the bony deformities and in planning for surgery.

In this patient, both ulcers healed when treated with thick felt deflections and lyofoam dressing. Other available treatments include Apligraft, a type of artificial skin to help with wound healing, or a total contact cast to redistribute weight-bearing and protect the ulcer.

Glycaemic control is very important in the treatment of diabetic ulcers. This patient, was in secondary failure and had a history of poor compliance, would benefit from having the different aspects of his diabetes managed in a single location such as a Diabetes Centre.

Learning points

This case illustrates how chronic poor control of diabetes can lead to neuropathic foot ulcers, which can become a long-term and major cause of morbidity. As with other diabetic complications, prevention is of the highest priority.

Chronic hyperglycaemia is the most important risk factor for diabetic neuropathy. One should aim for HbA1c concentrations of 7% or lower for ideal long-term control in order to reduce the development of diabetic complications including neuropathy. However, in the presence of coexistent diseases or advanced age this target would need to be appropriately adjusted in the individual patient. It is imperative to impress on the patient from the very first encounter the importance of their commitment to self-care. In many patients this requires considerable education, which is time-consuming. Thus all patients with newly diagnosed diabetes should be offered access to diabetes education.

Meticulous foot care is essential to prevent ulceration in patients with diabetic peripheral neuropathy, and often requires the help of family members. Regular and frequent reinforcement is important for diabetic self-care and optimization of diabetic management. Patients need to understand that the problem of neuropathic ulcer is prone to recur and that they need to seek help as soon as a problem is detected. The multidisciplinary input from the podiatrist, endocrinologist, diabetes educator and dietician available at Diabetes Centres is particularly valuable for this sort of patient.

Underlying bony deformities can cause neuropathic ulcers to recur. Early consultation with a specialist surgeon is worthwhile if deformities are marked, or if such an ulcer is slow to heal or recurs.

Suggested reading

Diabetes Control and Complications Trial Research Group. The effect of intensive diabetes therapy on the development and progression of neuropathy. *Ann Intern Med* 1995; 122: 561–8.

McNeely MJ, Boyko EJ, Ahroni JH et al. The independent contributions of diabetic neuropathy and vasculopathy in foot ulceration. How great are the risks? *Diabetes Care* 1995; 18: 216–19.

Pham H, Armstrong DG, Harvey C et al. Screening techniques to identify people at high risk for diabetic foot ulceration: a prospective multicenter trial. *Diabetes Care* 2000; 23: 606–11.

UK Prospective Diabetes Study Group. Intensive blood-glucose control with sulphonylureas or insulin compared with conventional treatment and risk of complications in patients with type 2 diabetes. *Lancet* 1998; 352: 837–53.

CASE 42: PYREXIA OF UNKNOWN ORIGIN?

Andrew JM Boulton

History

A 50-year-old Asian male was admitted as an emergency to a medical unit, with a 6-day history of fever and intermittent rigors. He had been diagnosed with type 2 diabetes 5 years previously whilst being investigated for sciatica and hypertension. At that time he was noted to have maculopathy, which was subsequently treated with laser therapy, proteinuria of 7 g/24 h, uncontrolled hypertension and sensory loss bilaterally below the knees. Despite triple therapy for hypertension, there was progressive loss of renal function, and for 12 months he had received continuous ambulatory peritoneal dialysis (CAPD) for renal failure. Medication on admission included: Mixtard 30/70 insulin b.d., enalapril, fusemide, one-alpha calcidol, aspirin and multiple vitamins.

Examination and investigations

The patient was pyrexial (38.6°C) and fluid-overloaded with bilateral ankle oedema. Blood pressure was 148/96 mmHg, heart sounds were normal. Bilateral basal crackles were noted on auscultation of the lungs. The abdomen was soft, and peritoneal dialysis (PD) fluid was clear and not clinically infected. No obvious cause of sepsis was noted on clinical examination.

Haemoglobin was 11.1 g%, the white cell count was 18.4×10^9/L. Blood cultures, PD fluid and catheter line cultures and MSSU were all negative. Chest X-ray showed cardiomegaly and early pulmonary oedema. Ultrasound exam of the abdomen revealed no obvious cause of sepsis.

Diagnosis

The initial diagnosis was pyrexia of unknown origin (PUO) in a type 2 diabetic patient on CAPD.

Treatment and outcome

Four days after admission a consultation to the diabetes team was requested. When I first examined the patient, I noted a dressing on his left great toe.

I enquired of the patient the indication for the dressing; he responded: 'As I told the other doctors, it is of no consequence: I simply cut myself when trimming my toe nail'. He was resistant to my suggestion that we remove the dressing, but eventually agreed. What lay beneath is shown in Figure 1: there was ulceration, gross infection and local cellulitis. I requested an urgent X-ray, a wound swab and a non-invasive vascular assessment. The X-ray of the foot revealed erosion of the distal phalanx compatible with osteomyelitis (Figure 2). Culture from the wound showed a heavy growth of *Staphylococcus aureus*. I recommended broad-spectrum antibiotics (ciproflaxacin 500 mg b.d. and clindamycin 150 mg qds) and an urgent surgical opinion for probable amputation of the great toe. The vascular assessment was satisfactory (no significant occlusive lesions) and the great toe was amputated. The wound was slow to heal and a further surgical debridement was required before the patient was eventually discharged home some weeks later.

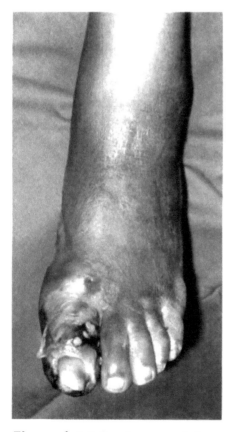

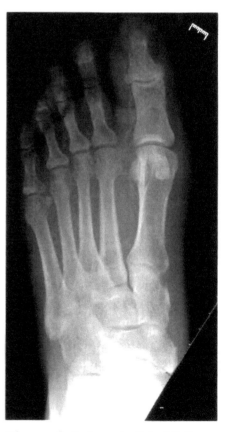

Figure 1 *Left foot showing marked sepsis associated with ulceration and desquamation of the great toe.*

Figure 2 *Radiograph of the left foot showing erosion of the terminal tuft of the great toe, especially medially, consistent with osteomyelitis. Note also extensive vascular calcification.*

Commentary

'For one mistake made for not knowing – ten mistakes are made for not looking'   (J. Lindsay)

This quotation, one of many adages by the late Professor Lindsay of Belfast, undoubtedly summarizes the management of this case. Throughout our medical training we are taught how to handle patients who present with symptoms and signs. Scant attention is paid to those who have no complaints because of sensory loss. Thus diabetic neuropathic patients with severe foot sepsis and even osteomyelitis or gangrene, may have no symptoms whatsoever,[1] and even suspecting a serious problem, are prone to minimize its seriousness.[2] On further questioning after discharge, the patient explained that 1 week before admission he had cut his toe badly whilst trimming his nails: it bled profusely, so he applied 'antiseptic' and put on a tight 'bandage' which he had not removed before admission. Had the patient presented to the foot clinic immediately after the injury, the admission and the amputation might have been prevented.

What did I learn from this case?

This case reinforces the need to assess the feet of every diabetic patient admitted to hospital for whatever reason – especially those known to have neuropathy. It also behoves us to emphasize the absolute requirement for regular foot inspection in diabetic patients not only to our junior staff, but also to medical and nursing students.

References

1. Jude EB, Boulton AJM. End-stage complications of diabetic neuropathy. *Diabetes Rev* 1999; **7**: 395–410.

2. Vileikyte L. Psychological and behavioural issues in diabetic neuropathic foot ulceration. In: Boulton AJM, Connor H, Cavanagh PR, eds. *The Foot in Diabetes*, 3rd edn. Chichester: J Wiley & Sons, 2000: 121–30.

Index